Contents

List of tables

Acknowledgements

The Research Unit of the Royal College of Physicians is supported by grants from the Wolfson Foundation, the Welton Foundation, PPP Medical Trust, and other charitable and research grants, along with a grant from the NHS Executive.

The West Midlands Geriatric Resource Centre is supported by the Academic Department of Geriatric Medicine of the University of Birmingham.

The authors are grateful to Isla Robert, Information Scientist at the West Midlands Geriatric Resource Centre, to colleagues who participated in the King's Fund/Audit Commission Joint Review Advisory Group, and to staff of the King's Fund Library.

Executive summary

Purpose and approach

This report presents the findings of a project that aimed to understand the present state of knowledge of the clinical effectiveness of rehabilitation using the evidence of systematic reviews. A systematic review is a formalised approach to identifying and synthesising the results of research studies, particularly controlled clinical trials. By using this approach, this report sought breadth of coverage to compare the effectiveness of rehabilitation in different situations in order to discern underlying principles and themes.

Definitions and tools

A working definition of rehabilitation was used, along with the conceptual framework of the International Classification of Impairment, Disability and Handicap. To these, three further tools were developed as part of the project – a classification of rehabilitation interventions, a classification of outcome measures and a draft prioritisation framework. These were used to describe and characterise in a systematic way the systematic reviews included in this report.

The systematic reviews

Fifty-six systematic reviews, covering a variety of disabilities, health problems, diseases and client groups were identified through a rigorous and comprehensive literature search. Data was extracted from them in a systematic way and is presented in full in this report as an evidence table.

The state of evidence

Topic coverage of the systematic reviews is not comprehensive and important gaps have been revealed. Further work is required to establish if these are gaps in the research base as well. Two main types of intervention have been evaluated – packages of care and simple interventions – but further important detail about components of the different interventions is often lacking. In addition, the use of outcome measures requires further development in order to allow easy pooling of the results of different trials and to take into account the different perspectives of the patient, carer and services.

Evidence of effective practice

There are positive results for the effectiveness of rehabilitation in a variety of key areas, which are discussed in detail, particularly when packages of care are used. Three examples are cardiac rehabilitation, stroke rehabilitation, and comprehensive geriatric assessment of older people. This trio may indicate the underlying need to co-ordinate and organise care when there are multiple risk factors to deal with, where multiple disciplines are involved in care, or where multiple phases of the rehabilitation process need to be considered (including access and assessment). They are complemented by positive results of patient education approaches which reflect the need for patient involvement and empowerment. The effect sizes that have been shown in these positive reviews are very large and exceed many of those seen with drug treatments. However, there is a lack of direct evidence about access and financing of rehabilitation.

The research base

Contrary to popular belief, a very large number of controlled trials of rehabilitation have been carried out. However, clear pointers as to how the quality of the research effort could be enhanced have emerged. These include a need for a transparent and workable priority setting system, standardisation of descriptions of interventions, introduction of a standard set of outcomes, along with increases in health economic input. Such changes might boost the profile and hence productivity of research in this area.

Recommendations

Suggestions for responding to the findings of this report are grouped into three categories of recommendations relating to: services now, future development and future research.

It is suggested that local services should respond to the needs of their local population, particularly those of older people, by facilitating access to rehabilitation through comprehensive assessment of individual need and through educational approaches that empower service users. Services should also be organised to achieve co-ordination of different interventions and different phases of the rehabilitation process.

Evidence from studies on cardiac rehabilitation, stroke rehabilitation and comprehensive geriatric assessment of older people should be translated into routine practice and used to inform rehabilitation developments for other conditions.

To implement these recommendations, a core set of generic tools and procedures is needed to facilitate the use of rehabilitative approaches in different settings (i.e. hospitals, care homes or private houses) – a service 'without walls'.

The future development of rehabilitation should be evaluated to strengthen the base of experience, knowledge and know-how. This would be best achieved through an existing quality improvement mechanism such as clinical audit. Further, a mechanism for cross learning is required so that important solutions to the organisation of complex rehabilitative care can be diffused easily through services. To foster greater uptake of knowledge, there should be closer liaison between research and routine care and a greater emphasis on training, education and team building.

Future research in rehabilitation will be required to fill gaps in knowledge and respond to the changing shape of services. Greater value will be obtained from the research effort using the measures described above. Greater harmonisation of outcome measurement and description of interventions will encourage further systematic reviews with even greater impact and meaning.

Conclusion

This report suggests that enough is now known from a clinical effectiveness perspective to move forward significantly in the organisation and provision of rehabilitation. Such is the scale of effects of rehabilitation that this would be expected to have a major impact on the state of services and the health of the population.

Chapter 1

Introduction

Key points

- A working definition of rehabilitation is being used which focuses on handicap.

- The International Classification of Impairment, Disability and Handicap provides a basic framework to consider health and rehabilitation which can be built upon to understand finer degrees of detail.

- Rehabilitation may comprise one or several inputs, take place in one or several types of settings and involve the patient in decision-making; these features mean it may be a challenging intervention to deliver effectively.

- Improving the quality of rehabilitation services requires information about clinical effectiveness.

- The clinical effectiveness and research base for rehabilitation is ill understood. This report focuses solely on the evidence from systematic reviews.

Overview

This report presents an analysis of present understanding of the clinical effectiveness of rehabilitation based solely on the evidence of published systematic reviews of the literature. This report was commissioned jointly by the King's Fund and the Audit Commission as part of their work of appraising the current status of and knowledge about the rehabilitation of adults who have been disabled by illness or injury. The overall focus of this work included access, organisation, therapeutic intervention, cost and modes of financing. This clinical effectiveness report has been produced in parallel with a report on policy developments and trends in rehabilitation which has been carried out by the Social Policy Research Unit of the University of York.

What is rehabilitation?

For the purpose of this report, the King's Fund define rehabilitation as:

> a process aiming to restore personal autonomy in those aspects of daily living considered most relevant by patients or service users, and their family carers.

This is a working approach with an emphasis on handicap. It is recognised that there are many definitions of rehabilitation and that no single definition is universally accepted. Indeed, some would argue that rehabilitation is too complex a concept, process or activity to define to the satisfaction of all agencies. A useful description of the role of rehabilitation, which echoes the importance of considering handicap, has been provided:

Rehabilitation should aim to maximise the patient's role fulfilment and independence in his/her environment, all within the limitations imposed by the underlying pathology and impairments and by the availability of resources. This helps the person to make the best adaptation possible to any difference between roles achieved and roles desired. [Wade DT, 1992]

Rehabilitation and health

Whatever definition is adopted, rehabilitation is intimately tied up with processes which act at multiple levels in the hierarchy of health. These can be considered using the International Classification of Impairment, Disability and Handicap. Rehabilitation is relevant to interventions which act upon disrupted physiology and pathology in organs affected by disease and age – the *impairment* level. It may also be directed at improving the functioning of the individual – the *disability* level. Finally, there may be the ultimate aim to enhance social role functioning as indicated in the preceding description – the *handicap* level. This linked hierarchy is illustrated in Table 1. Not only does this simple framework help understanding of the nature of rehabilitative interventions but it also provides a reminder of the wide spectrum of appropriate outcomes of rehabilitation that might need to be considered.

Table 1 The International Classification of Impairment, Disability and Handicap in action

Health Level	Explanation	Example
Impairment	Disrupted physiology and pathology in organs affected by disease and age	Osteoarthritis of the knee
Disability	Reduction in the functional status of the individual	Difficulty in walking
Handicap	Effect on social role function	Unable to go to the supermarket to shop

Rehabilitation as an intervention

Rehabilitation is a continuous and multifactorial process which is often dependent on multiple inputs. Because of this, rehabilitation requires a range of skills and expertise that is not usually available from one individual. This often means that a team delivers rehabilitation with a task and goal-oriented approach. In addition, as health care becomes a community-oriented activity (rather than one centred around secondary care hospitals), there may be the challenge of power shifting more to patients and carers and away from the professional [Keir D, 1996]. Thus, one might consider that rehabilitation might make particular demands of co-ordination, organisation and communication. These demands will inevitably influence the future process and organisation of rehabilitation. For example, an intervention which is applied across several sectors of care will provoke considerable challenges in relation to clinical records, continuity of care and seamless delivery. Overall, therefore, rehabilitation is often a complex intervention whether one is considering the inputs, the role of the user or the challenges to high quality care.

Clinical effectiveness and quality improvement

This report concentrates on clinical effectiveness with an eye towards quality improvement to reflect growing trends in the service. This is defined as:

the extent to which specific clinical interventions when deployed in the field for a particular patient or population, do what they are intended to do – i.e. maintain and improve health and secure the greatest possible health gain from the available resources. [NHS Executive 1996]

Thus, the focus of this report is on an understanding of the evidence of published research in order that it can be put into routine clinical practice. This is the first stage towards high quality services which should be based on doing 'the right things . . . well' [Hopkins 1990].

The content boundaries

The boundaries of rehabilitation are fuzzy and so a wide approach to content has been adopted to reflect the broad nature of rehabilitation. In general, the coverage of this report is over-inclusive. The term clinical is used in its widest sense to include a range of interventions which might or might not improve health through rehabilitation. Although such interventions might include a social care element, the focus is not on purely social or economic interventions that might improve health, but excludes those that are not primarily rehabilitative in nature. Thus, for example, this report would include a review of community health team management aimed at improving handicap levels which included social work input. It would include a review of day services showing how social service staff rehabilitate people in their own home after hip fracture. However, a review of a purely social intervention such as increasing child benefit to improve the diet of schoolchildren would not.

Pressures around rehabilitation and research

This snapshot of current knowledge of the clinical effectiveness of rehabilitation is taken at a time when there are many forces acting on the future of rehabilitation. These factors include the trend to community-based health care, the interest in extending the quality of life of the population, the economic pressure of long-term care, changes in specialist professional activity and the influence of the NHS internal market. These forces are becoming bound together by the growing interest in quality improvement and clinical effectiveness as integrating forces in the NHS. In many respects the expectations of rehabilitation are becoming higher and may be moving at a faster pace than the research effort. Yet, paradoxically, rehabilitation services are under threat as commissioners of health care increasingly require supportive evidence of clinical effectiveness before contracting for services. Several factors contribute to this threat, including the belief that rehabilitation has a weak evidence base to support it. Certainly research in rehabilitation has traditionally been considered difficult with little hope of funding. In addition, long-held views such as 'rehabilitation belongs to therapists' have implied that rehabilitation is distinct from medicine and consequently inferior to it. This creates uncertainty about the role and place of rehabilitation in modern health care delivery, which may be exacerbated by the low public appeal for a 'low-tech' type of health care.

Using systematic reviews to understand rehabilitation effectiveness

There have been few attempts to summarise the effectiveness of rehabilitation based on empirical findings. Some have used traditional reviews but this approach has several limitations. First, such reviews may be biased because of the pre-existing views or interests of the author. Second, identification of the literature may be incomplete. Third, the likely effect on practice is uncertain; strongly positive or negative results may be dismissed as biased; inconclusive results are unhelpful in decision-making. Systematic reviews are a method which may help to resolve these inconsistencies. They demand a much more transparent approach to all aspects of reviewing – systematic literature searching, quality assessment of reports and pooling of quantitative results (such as by formal meta-analysis). The importance of this approach is now clearly recognised and has been adopted and promoted by the Cochrane Collaboration [Cochrane Collaboration 1997], the Effective Health Care Bulletin programme [NHS CRD 1996] and the Health Technology Assessment programme [NHS Executive 1997]. It identifies consistencies and inconsistencies between the results of typically under-powered trials. In this report we present a summary of systematic reviews of rehabilitation in order to understand this body of evidence, while recognising that there will be areas where systematic reviews have not been carried out although primary research results do exist.

Structure of this report

This report first presents the methods that were used to identify interventions, outcomes and published systematic reviews. This leads to a detailed description of the findings, which are presented in three parts – findings relating to methodology, those relating to the quality and coverage of the systematic reviews and those reporting what the systematic reviews show. A series of tables is provided to complement a large, comprehensive evidence table which presents all the key characteristics and results of the included systematic reviews. These findings are then discussed within the present and future context of the UK's health and community care services, leading to a series of recommendations before final conclusions are drawn.

Chapter 2

Methods

Key points

- A method to describe the components of a spectrum of interventions from different perspectives was developed.

- An inventory of different outcomes measures and a means to classify them was developed.

- Candidate reviews were identified through a wide search of electronic bibliographic databases, hand-searching and appeals for information.

- Systematic reviews were selected and data extracted from them in a standardised fashion.

- An approach to prioritising topics for systematic reviews was developed.

Overview

Rehabilitation covers a diverse range of activities. Therefore an approach was developed to capture a broad range of interventions, outcomes and sources of reviews. Since no single definition is accepted for clinical, scientific or indexing purposes, this approach needed to acquire a wide range of evidence of clinical effectiveness. This section describes how this was done as a 'systematic overview' of systematic reviews.

Identifying the spectrum of interventions

In order to conduct a thorough search, a standard way of describing rehabilitation interventions was created from an inventory of possible criteria. A draft inventory was generated through a discussion with a multidisciplinary Disability Focus Group at Selly Oak Hospital, Birmingham. This was refined and amended by the authors and through discussion with the Joint Advisory Group of the King's Fund and the Audit Commission. To gain greater understanding of the user perspective on this subject the concept of rehabilitation was also discussed with a sample of in-patients in Birmingham. Most people had little idea what rehabilitation meant. To some, rehabilitation referred to young people recovering from road accidents and to employment. Few thought it was a clear part of the health service. However, many were familiar with one of the key stages of rehabilitation, assessment, through personal experience.

Identifying measures of outcome

A wide range of possible outcomes of rehabilitation is possible, but a method of assessing the systematic reviews was needed. A classification system was therefore developed in the following manner. The lists of outcomes were taken from the reports of three user-focused national workshops which had been held for clinical guideline development. These were synthesised and categorised for discussion at a local level and by the Joint Advisory group of the King's Fund and the Audit Commission.

Identifying candidate reviews

A multipronged approach was taken to identifying candidate reviews. A range of potential sources was identified – public publications databases, an in-house database of clinical effectiveness, the national Clinical Guidelines Register in the Health Care of Older People, *Current Medical Literature – Health Care of Older People*, and original journals. In addition, we obtained subject lists from the Chartered Society of Physiotherapy. Table 2 summarises the scope of the search. These information resources were searched using predefined search strategies as outlined below and shown in Appendices 1 and 2.

Table 2 Scope of the literature search

Broad category	Details
Literature databases	Cochrane Library (contains a number of databases) MEDLINE NHS Economic Evaluation Database (NEED) Psych Lit Social Science Citation Index CINAHL
Other bibliography	National clinical guideline register Clinical effectiveness bibliography of the Research Unit, RCP
Journals etc.	*Current Medical Literature (Health Care of Older People)* *Age and Ageing* *Journal of the American Geriatrics Society*
Appeal	*Linker* R&D newsletter

Publications databases

The following literature databases were searched:

Cochrane Library: this contains a number of databases of systematic and other reviews. The software for this database is evolving and it was not possible to search precisely for topics without incurring a lot of irrelevant material.

MEDLINE: this is the primary publications database for the medical literature. It includes indexed entries from many journals and can be searched using sophisticated methods. The search strategy used was designed to find as precisely as possible systematic reviews including meta-analysis on rehabilitation, using the search strategy of the Centre for Reviews and Dissemination. This uses MeSH (subject headings) and free text with truncation to maximise the precision of the search. It excludes publication types: review, multicase, and review of reported cases. This produces the maximum numbers of systematic reviews that have been indexed by MEDLINE. The search was carried out for the period 1966–96.

NHS Economic Evaluation Database (NEED): this database is produced by the Centre for Reviews and Dissemination (CRD) focusing on economic evaluation of health care. These reviews are therefore different from systematic reviews but it was searched in case some of the subjects matched up with systematic reviews and in so doing provided us with both clinical effectiveness and cost effectiveness information.

Psych LIT: this indexes the professional and academic literature in psychology and related disciplines. The search engine is not as precise as that of MEDLINE so the term 'overview' was included in order to identify systematic reviews for the period 1984–96.

Social Sciences Citation Index: this database indexes core journals in the social sciences, education, law, management, philosophy, and psychology. It is not very precise for searching for systematic reviews because of limitations in the search engine. The term 'overview' was used as an additional search item. The search covered 1984–96.

CINAHL: the Nursing and Allied Health (CINAHL) database provides comprehensive coverage of the English language journal literature for nursing and allied health disciplines. Material from over 950 journals is included in CINAHL, covering health education, occupational therapy, physical therapy, and social sciences. As with several of the other databases, it is difficult to identify systematic reviews because CINAHL does not have a publication type – meta-analysis. Thus, the term overview was substituted.

Other sources

Clinical Guidelines Register (Health Care of Older People): this register contains about 1500 national clinical guidelines and policy documents produced in the UK. Relevant publications were inspected for potential inclusion in this review.

Clinical effectiveness bibliography of the Research Unit, Royal College of Physicians: this contains about 5000 citations of published papers on clinical effectiveness. The bibliography was searched electronically using customised key words.

Current Medical Literature – Health Care of Older People: this is a quarterly publication which presents short reviews of selected publications concerned with the health care of older people. About 400 papers are reviewed each year. Selections are taken from a quarterly literature search of a wide range of journals as indicated in Appendix 3. This publication was checked for reviews published during the last five years.

Handsearching: two publications – *Age and Ageing* and *Journal of the American Geriatrics Society* – were handsearched for reviews published during the last five years.

Appeal: An appeal for information about unpublished or recently completed research projects was published in the Spring edition of *Linker*, the newsletter of the National R&D Network in the Health Care of Older People (circulation about 6,500).

Selecting reviews for the overview

A large number of reviews of rehabilitation were identified through this search strategy and were considered for inclusion. The electronic records of candidate reviews were assessed on the initial selection sieve. Full hard copies of reviews were obtained and those for inclusion in this report were selected. The key features for the systematic reviews were: defining the topic of interest, identifying trials systematically and examining their quality. Many of the systematic reviews also contain a quantitative pooling of the findings of the primary research studies (known as meta-analysis).

Data extraction

Information was extracted from the reviews in a standard fashion using an evidence table which is described in greater detail in the next section. One report author carried out the data extraction initially and this was then checked by the other report author. Any differences of opinion were discussed and resolved.

A framework for priorities

In order to assess the present coverage of systematic reviews, rules for judging the importance of topics were developed. A large number of potential criteria were discussed and matches were then sought with a variety of key points to build a working framework.

Chapter 3

Findings – methodology

Key points

- A comprehensive standardised description of a rehabilitation intervention will include the following criteria – study population, purpose, nature, staff, setting and timing.

- There are many options for these criteria, which means that rehabilitation interventions may vary considerably in their nature and components but can still be described.

- The classification of outcome measures is broken into three main categories – patient-oriented outcomes (including impairment outcomes, disability outcomes and handicap outcomes), carer-oriented outcomes and service-oriented outcomes.

- Priorities for understanding the clinical effectiveness of rehabilitation can be constructed according to several dimensions such as population burden, patients' values, carers' perspectives, service measures and policy emphasis.

Overview

This section presents the first set of findings relating to the methodological clarification of interventions, outcomes and priorities.

Identifying the spectrum of interventions

A standard description of interventions was developed that uses six headings. Appendix 4 shows the details. This attempts to provide a framework to classify rehabilitation interventions by defining:

The study population: the subjects for whom the interventions are intended.

Purpose: why the intervention is being delivered and/or evaluated.

Nature: the intervention or package of interventions that is being evaluated.

Staff: the personnel who are responsible for or involved in the delivery of the intervention. This may include medical, nursing and therapy staff. In a team package of care, other disciplines may be important too. It may also include non-clinical staff such as managers, social workers and others. Other personnel such as complementary practitioners and lay people may also be involved.

Setting: where the intervention is being delivered. This may vary from hospital or community settings. The former may include tertiary care, general hospitals, community hospitals and specialist in-patient services (such as rehabilitation units or centres). In the community setting, the study population may receive the intervention in their own home, in a long-term care facility or at a centre which is attended such as a day centre, or primary health care facility.

Timing: the timing of the use of the intervention in relation to the original event that led to the need for rehabilitation. This may be in the acute, post-acute or chronic phase of care. The definition of the timing of care may also be related to transitions in care, such as discharge from hospital or long-term care entry.

Wide range of possible interventions

Although a wide range of rehabilitation interventions is possible, this classification allows for a standard description of a very large number of combinations. A second advantage of this approach is that it maintains broad awareness of many different aspects of rehabilitation. For example, assessment is the key to determining the correct intervention to be used. This involves a multiprofessional approach to defining what disabilities are present and their causes or contributing factors, planning interventions to minimise disability and handicap, setting goals with the other, determining a prognosis, and establishing a way to monitor progress.

Identifying measures of outcome

A working classification was developed and the results are shown in Appendix 5. The main feature of this inventory is to break outcomes into three main groups – patient-oriented, carer-oriented and service-oriented outcomes. Of these groups, the largest number of well-recognised measures is in the patient-oriented category, but this may partly reflect lack of agreement on typology for the other categories.

Patient-oriented outcomes

Patient-oriented outcomes are broken down into seven categories. The first three are: Impairment, Disability and Handicap, defined as discussed, by the International Classification of Impairment, Disability and Handicap. The next category concerns morbidity and mortality. Pain, such a prominent aspect of many chronic disabling conditions, is singled out as a separate category as is patient satisfaction. An 'other' category is included as a catch-all.

Towards priorities on rehabilitation evidence

Table 3 shows the criteria that could be used to understand the adequacy of coverage of knowledge about rehabilitation. From a population point of view, leading causes of disability (such as arthritis) or lost work (from back pain) would be seen as important. From a patient perspective, falls or incontinence would be important. From a carer perspective, immobility or 'challenging' behaviour in Alzheimer's disease might emerge as priority areas. Consideration from a service perspective could be based on costs and/or

Table 3 Approaches to prioritisation in rehabilitation and review coverage

Source of priority	Examples	Source of data to assess importance
Patient	Falls Immobility Off legs Incontinence Mental illness Addictions Arthritis Coronary artery disease Chest disease	User groups General Household Survey Patient Charter Information
Carer	Need for support Alzheimer's disease	Carers' and relatives' groups
Service	Bed blocking Hip fracture Stroke	Volumes and costs Professional and other related organisations
Population	Disabling conditions	OPCS Disability survey 'Burden' models Public health dataset Outcome indicators
Policy	NHS medium-term priorities Health of the Nation Perceived pressures (such as winter bed pressures)	Routine data

volume and might include minor psychological problems or fractured neck of femur. Debate may be needed to bring together these perspectives and reach common understanding with research funding bodies.

Chapter 4

Findings – quality and coverage

Key points

- The presented evidence table shows key information about the reviews included in this report covering general characteristics, classification of intervention, classification of outcomes and findings.

- Topic coverage in the systematic reviews has not been comprehensive. This may reflect gaps in systematic reviews, primary research or both along with a possible failure to capture all relevant information, particularly that which is unpublished.

- The two main types of intervention are complex packages of care and simpler, often unitary, interventions.

- Information is scant about the purpose, staffing and timing of interventions.

- A comprehensive and unified approach to the use of outcomes measures appears to be lacking and may hamper meaningful aggregation for meta-analysis.

Overview

This section describes in detail the quality of the systematic reviews included in this report. These are listed in the evidence table and key aspects are discussed in a series of subsections.

The evidence table – overview

A comprehensive distillation of the reviews appears in the evidence table (Appendix 6), which shows the characteristics and findings of the reviews. As this is a large table, a word of explanation and orientation is appropriate. Each row comprises a single report identified by the authors. There are then four groups of columns: I – Report Characteristics, II – Description of intervention, III – Outcomes used, and IV – Findings.

I – Report Characteristics: this presents, in order, the names of the authors, the year of publication, the country of origin, the type of review, the trials used and the study population. In describing the type of review we have used three terms: *meta-analysis* refers to a systematic review with statistical pooling of results which is published in a recognised journal; *Cochrane Reviews* refers to a systematic review with statistical pooling of results which has been performed to the standards of the Cochrane Collaboration and is published in the Cochrane Library; *systematic review* refers to a review based on a systematic search of the literature but not including statistical pooling of results. It should be noted that *country of origin* refers to the source of the review itself rather than the source of all the constituent trials which may be drawn from a much wider geographical area.

II – Description of intervention: this includes a breakdown of the characteristics of the intervention according to the classification described in the previous section.

III – Outcomes used: this includes a breakdown of the outcomes used according to the classification described in the previous section.

IV – Findings: where available this indicates the results of statistical pooling, along with the authors' conclusions and a comment.

Study populations

The concentration of attention in the reviews has been on a relatively limited number of situations, as indicated in Table 4. This apparent bias may be because of the real lack of primary research or may simply reflect the interests of the research and review community. Of the client groups, research concerned with the care of people with mental illness has appeared most. No problem of disability stands out apart from back/spinal pain. Of the diseases, most reviews have considered stroke and ischaemic heart disease. Little work appears to have been done on several important problems that might be defined as priorities from the standpoints such as those described above. However, the primary literature needs to be searched to establish whether these gaps are present in the research effort too.

Table 4 Main situations subjected to systematic review

Broad focus	Detailed topic	Number of reports
Client group	People with mental illness/psychological concerns	4
	Surgical patients	3
	Need for rehabilitation/disabled people	2
	Older people	2
Problem/disability	Musculoskeletal disease	1
	Back and spinal pain	10
	Alcohol misuse	2
	Aphasia	2
	Incontinence	1
	Falls	1
Disease	Stroke	8
	Coronary artery disease	7
	Chronic obstructive pulmonary disease	3
	Asthma	1
	Diabetes	2
	Hip fracture	1
	Other	6

Purpose

No reports appear to be explicit about the purpose of the intervention and so this criterion has been excluded from the evidence table. In many cases the purpose is implicit in the description of the intervention but this is not always the case.

Table 5 Broad aspects of intervention subjected to review, using intervention classification

Broad focus	Type of intervention	Number of reports
Purpose		0
Nature of intervention	Simple therapy/physical	24
	Multiple intervention packages/interprofessional	16
	General rehabilitation	8
	Simple psychosocial/educational	4
	Simple medical	3
	Unclear/mixed	2
Setting	Hospital	11
	Mixed	10
	Community care	2
	Primary care	1
	Interface	1
	Unclear	31
Timing phase	Post acute	15
	Mixed	4
	Perioperative	2
	Unclear	35

Intervention types

There were two large groups of intervention types (as shown in Table 5). The largest group covered simple interventions such as physiotherapy, exercise or TENS (trans-cutaneous electrical nervous stimulation) [24/56]. The next largest group [16/56] was concerned with various multiple intervention packages and trials of co-ordination, teams and interprofessional working. There was a small number of reports of simple medical, psychosocial or educational interventions.

Staff

Very little information is provided about the staff involved in these interventions. In some cases, such as a review of occupational therapy, this may be surmised but in general little information is presented about the personnel. A notable exception is the most recent systematic review of stroke unit care [Stroke Unit Trialists 1997b].

Setting

Rather surprisingly, the setting of care is poorly presented in these reviews, as shown in Table 5. Where the setting of care is clear, in-patient hospital sites and mixed sites predominate.

Timing/phase

Similarly there is little explicit detail about the timing of interventions. Again, assumptions can be made in some cases. When articulated, the post-acute phase of care was the commonest.

Table 6 Outcomes used in the reviewed literature

Focus	Domain	Number of studies
Patient orientation	Impairment	40
	Disability	25
	Handicap (incl. work, mood, QoL)	20
	Morbidity/mortality	15
	Pain	11
	Service satisfaction	4
	Goal attainment	0
	Other	26
Carer orientation	Carer strain/health	3
	Satisfaction	1
Service orientation	Service use	8
	Length of stay	8
	Institutionalisation/place of domicile/discharge	5
	Cost	3
	Other	5

Outcomes used

A wide range of outcomes has been used in the reported studies, covering the three main categories and most domains of the classification of outcomes, as shown in Table 6. However, there is great unevenness and inappropriateness in the application of outcome measures. From the patient orientation, measures of impairment tend to dominate along with a group of miscellaneous measures. This means that much of the effectiveness of rehabilitation is being judged in a way that may not be directly related to the goals that it is seeking to achieve. For example, cardiac rehabilitation may be judged according to an outcome such as the presence of high blood pressure (an impairment) whereas the level of consequent disability may be more relevant. Measures of disability appear in under half of reviews. Handicap measures are similarly represented when measures of quality of life are included under this heading. Morbidity and mortality feature in about a third of reports, along with pain. Satisfaction rarely appears and goal attainment is not encountered. Carer outcomes are very rarely mentioned. Service outcomes are surprisingly little used, concentrating on length of hospital stay. Costing and health economics are very weak. Overall, no studies appear to report the use of a full range of appropriate outcomes across the classification of outcomes.

Chapter 5

Findings – what the systematic reviews show

Key points

- Many of the systematic reviews of rehabilitation present positive evidence of clinical effectiveness but a significant number, particularly those involving simple interventions, present equivocal or negative results.

- Important positive findings include those concerned with cardiac and stroke rehabilitation, and comprehensive assessment of older people. These suggest that effective rehabilitation may be achieved by the co-ordination of complex interventions addressing multiple risk factors, involving multiple professional disciplines and multiple phases of rehabilitation.

- Positive findings also include educational approaches to care, illustrating the importance of patient empowerment in rehabilitation.

- There is a lack of direct information about access and financing of care.

- The status of rehabilitation research is mixed; on the one hand a very large number of trials have been carried out; on the other hand, the quality and methodology may be inadequate for modern health services.

Overview

This section presents in detail the findings of the systematic reviews. This is done in two main ways: first, there is discussion from the perspective of different clinical topics such as stroke, back pain etc; second, the results are considered in relation to the type of intervention and system issues such as co-ordination, access and organisation.

Significant results

Overall, many reviews present positive findings of the clinical effectiveness of the interventions under review. Thus, review evidence has been published which is broadly in favour of rehabilitation interventions for:

- a range of problems – including back pain and incontinence
- a range of diagnoses – including diabetes, chronic respiratory disease, coronary artery disease and stroke
- a range of client groups – including frail older people, people with mental health problems and surgical patients
- a range of types of interventions – including assessment and family therapy.

There are, however, a number of reviews with negative or equivocal results. Negative results, providing no evidence of effectiveness, apply to single interventions such as biofeedback in stroke (a means of developing awareness of breathing patterns and pulse rates and undertaking exercises to restore them to normal), case management and liaison in mental health, exercise in coronary artery disease, laser, ultrasound and biofeedback treatments. The review of care for people with fractured neck of femur is equivocal, providing inconsistent evidence of effectiveness. This is also true of reviews of speech and language therapy, falls prevention and some of those of physiotherapy. Some reviews (for example that of occupational therapy) appear to be inappropriately enthusiastic about the benefits.

Stroke rehabilitation

Of particular significance to future service developments are the reviews of co-ordinated stroke rehabilitation. They report broadly consistent results, using overlapping groups of studies, when considering package, team and co-ordination approaches to rehabilitation. The underlying theme appears to be the proper organisation of care to meet the needs of a particular client group. The most recent review [Stroke Unit Trialists 1997b] has revealed the importance of different features of the intervention, such as co-ordinated multidisciplinary care, education and training and specialisation of staff. Thus, stroke care may be an appropriate model for understanding the efficacy of rehabilitation in other situations when the linking and co-ordination of several inputs is required.

Cardiac rehabilitation

There are significant positive results in the area of cardiac rehabilitation. The relevance of these is threefold: first there is a key link between the secondary prevention of disease and rehabilitation which is not always emphasised; second, these results highlight the potential role of lifestyle change in rehabilitation, in this case around the modification of risk factors for coronary artery disease; third, there is an indication of opportunities for rehabilitative approaches to care. In this case, the patient has been through a recent life-threatening situation and motivation to participate may be elevated. Thus, cardiac rehabilitation may be a model for a situation where there are multiple risk factors, all of a different nature, to be tackled. However, studies in predominantly older subjects are still relatively lacking, which is an important omission.

Assessment and rehabilitation in general

There are two reviews which look at the general aspects of rehabilitation and both are positive. Of greatest interest is the systematic review of comprehensive geriatric assessment where the results indicate a major effect in a variety of settings even when the recommendations of the assessment were not controlled. Since assessment is a key stage of rehabilitation, upon which is based subsequent management, the significance of this review cannot be underestimated. Comprehensive geriatric assessment was generally a systematic process, carried out by an interdisciplinary team, in order to identify impairments and disabilities, particularly in relation to common challenges such as falls, immobility, cognitive impairment, and incontinence. This particular review may indicate the importance of the different phases of the rehabilitation process and of the role of assessment in recognising the need for and organisation of a complex approach to care.

Back pain

There is a large number of reviews on the subject of back pain. The results of these are mixed in relation to manipulation and physiotherapy but are positive about TENS. The use of ultrasound appears to be ineffective. Back pain is of major importance to the workforce and so the role of rehabilitation may require closer examination.

Other packages

The evidence around fractured neck of femur is equivocal. This may reflect the relatively small number of studies and the diversity of the actual interventions delivered. However, the evidence around enhanced peri-operative care (i.e. before, during and after operations) is encouraging. Mental health interventions show mixed effectiveness; there is particular controversy about case management and the result of the review appears to conflict with policy. Yet, closer examination of the review reveals diverse study populations. Family therapy for schizophrenia appears favourable.

Educational approaches

In two chronic disease situations, diabetes and chronic obstructive airways disease, educational approaches have been effective. These are relevant as they indicate the potential role for the patient in rehabilitation and coincide with the general theme of patient empowerment. This is supported further by the positive review of peri-operative care.

Simple interventions

In general, the evidence from these systematic reviews tends not to support simple and single interventions. The reason for this contrast with complex interventions is discussed below.

Access

There is no explicit information about altering access to rehabilitation. However, the trials of comprehensive geriatric assessment indicate that this may be an important part of effective delivery since it leads to identification of remediable problems, opening doors to therapeutic intervention. Moreover, the reviews indicate a role for improving access at all stages of care through patient education and empowerment.

Organisation and complexity

There is positive evidence for the organisation of complex care from the work on stroke, cardiac rehabilitation and comprehensive geriatric assessment. However, there is uncertainty about which component of organisation is important as the inputs are generally not well described. This criticism applies to many of the multifactorial interventions. Complex interventions seem more efficacious than single interventions. For example:

- Cardiac rehabilitation as compared with exercise alone
- Chronic obstructive pulmonary disease care as compared with isolated components of care in this area
- Stroke unit care as compared with individual therapies

Since complex interventions require some degree of organisation simply to deliver them, a service organisation is clearly important. This would apply to stroke and cardiac rehabilitation, and comprehensive geriatric assessment and others. Thus, the organisation of complex interventions may be highly relevant to effective rehabilitation; the more one can achieve co-ordination of diverse inputs through a systematic approach, protocol or team delivery the more effective the rehabilitation may be. There are three possible explanations: organisation and co-ordination may allow the additive effects of individually weak interventions to be seen. Further, organisation and co-ordination may allow synergy between different inputs; finally, organisation and co-ordination may provide a setting for goal setting, training and specialisation which may be prerequisites for success.

Effect sizes

The argument in favour of additive or synergistic effects may be based on the effect sizes that are seen. In stroke unit care, there were very large reductions in adverse outcomes: 28% reduction in death, 25% reduction in death/institutionalisation and 29% reduction in death/dependence. The 'numbers needed to treat' to avoid one adverse outcome were 22, 14 and 16 respectively and are at a level which has real importance for a local service. If the effect sizes for comprehensive geriatric assessment are considered then a similar picture emerges: a 35% reduction in death rate and a 12% reduction in subsequent admissions to hospital. Effect sizes of this magnitude are greater than those seen for many accepted drug treatments. This may also provide an explanation for the negative results for simple interventions if the effect size due to them is small when they are used alone. This may mean that testing the effectiveness of single interventions may need very large trials (which may be impractical) or that they should be included in factorial research designs within packages of care.

Financing of care

There are no reviews covering different models of financing care.

Status of rehabilitation research

Analysing these published systematic reviews sheds some light on the quality and status of rehabilitation research. Although a common assertion is that there is little rehabilitation research, the reviews presented are based on a very large number of controlled clinical trials which included very many subjects. These reviews focus on controlled clinical trials, mainly randomised trials and many of the reviews indicate the large number of other studies of weaker design which were found but rejected from the review process. Problems exist with definitions of rehabilitation, defining the intervention, the power of studies, the matching of studies to priority service issues and the appropriate use of outcome measures. It is difficult to conduct research on rehabilitation due to the lack of

Table 7 Systematic review. A '3' indicates that a systematic review has been carried out

Proposed priority category	Proposed priority area	Single intervention	Complex intervention	Service package
Problems	Falls and accidents	✓		
	Immobility			
	Off-legs			
	Incontinence	✓		
	Iatrogenesis			
Diseases	Mental illness		✓	✓
	Addictions			
	Arthritis			
	Coronary artery disease		✓	
	Chest disease		✓	
	Alzheimer's disease			
	Hip fracture			✓
	Stroke	✓	✓	✓
Service policy	Bed blocking			

researchers, definitional uncertainty, methodological challenges, and the heterogeneity of subject populations. Thus, it is not surprising that there are important gaps in current knowledge. We have already touched upon an approach to prioritising research topics (Table 3). Table 7 develops this theme further by considering a range of topics and showing whether a review exists or not.

Chapter 6

Discussion

Key points

- Systematic reviews point to the effectiveness of rehabilitation for a range of key mainstream topics despite the lack of a comprehensive portfolio of evidence.

- Generic themes underlying the positive reviews revolve around the organisation of complex interventions whether that complexity is derived from multiple areas for intervention (the multiple risk factors of cardiac rehabilitation), multiple inputs (the multidisciplinary roles in stroke rehabilitation) or multiple tasks (the multiple domains of assessment in comprehensive geriatric assessment).

- Since all disease processes can result in disability and handicap, an understanding of the balance of effectiveness between generic interventions and specific interventions will be needed.

- There are important limitations to the evidence in relation to health economics, research methodology, and the roles of social and environmental interventions.

- The research portfolio could be especially strengthened by listing priorities, encouraging community-based work, standardising descriptions of interventions, agreeing a comprehensive range of outcomes, and developing an appraisal of health economics.

Overview

This overview of reviews has revealed some important insights into the future role and development of rehabilitation. Overall, there is evidence of the clinical effectiveness of a range of rehabilitative interventions in a variety of conditions. This appears to be particularly relevant when the style of intervention matches the condition in question. For example, the most positive results for stroke care are related to the co-ordination of multiprofessional input, and this principle appears to apply to other situations. First, we present as the core of the report, our findings about the effectiveness of rehabilitation. We then discuss the limitations of the evidence. We end with recommendations about implementation of service delivery, research and development.

The clinical effectiveness of rehabilitation

Effectiveness in general: there is evidence of effectiveness in a number of disease and problem areas that are of high relevance to the health service, the population, individuals and their families. However, the size of the benefit or gain in health status was often relatively limited. This was compounded by weaknesses in methodology and coverage as discussed below.

Specific health areas: there appears to be good evidence of effectiveness for cardiac rehabilitation, organised stroke care, and comprehensive geriatric assessment. Educational approaches to cardiac rehabilitation appear to be high on the list for implementation, along with incontinence and possibly falls, and fractured neck of femur. However, there was a lack of comprehensive coverage of reviews for a wide range of common health problems such as osteoporosis, pressure sores and hypertension.

Generic themes: each area where rehabilitation appears to be effective discloses an underlying theme that may be of relevance to other areas. Since rehabilitation involves multiple inputs for agreed objectives, it is not surprising that the generic themes of organisation, co-ordination and interdisciplinary working appear to emerge.

- *Tackling known multiple risk factors* The evidence around cardiac rehabilitation may demonstrate a general message about tackling multiple risk factors in the prevention of further disease. This may point to the potential for a basic rehabilitation approach to other conditions which share multiple risk factors such as stroke. Rehabilitation may also include those changes in behaviour and lifestyle which can manifest or prevent certain risk factors from developing, such as exercise. Falls prevention is another condition for which there is a well-established risk factor profile which could be amenable to rehabilitation by reducing prescriptions for sedative drugs, for example or training to improve balance.
- *Co-ordinating various disciplines* The findings about stroke rehabilitation may apply to areas where several disciplines have a distinctive and complementary role and to similar situations such as the management of other disabling conditions. This will be especially applicable where the disabilities are similar as in the case of severe osteoarthritis or Parkinson's disease since the interventions may be comparable but not necessarily identical. Where the disability is different the rehabilitation approach will also be different and findings cannot be generalised. These reviews also fail in general to discuss what methods were used to enhance or maintain effective communication and co-ordination between the disciplines.
- *Access to the phases of rehabilitation* The review of comprehensive geriatric assessment may conceal a wider message about systematic approaches to accessing rehabilitation and other interventions through assessment pathways. Little information is available on the role of easy access to rehabilitation care (geographic distance to rehabilitation centre or staff availability) by comparison with difficult access. This area has profound importance for disabled and older people who might prefer community-based rehabilitation approaches and more individual attention rather than secondary care-based approaches.
- *Common effects* One must also bear in mind that the aim of rehabilitation is to reduce disability and handicap. Since there is a limited way in which disability may be expressed, techniques and programmes used for specific diseases may work on generic issues such as daily living (bathing, feeding, dressing, etc). Thus, there may be opportunities for cross learning in the organisation and delivery of services.

Simple or complex interventions: although rehabilitation usually means working with a team of trained professionals, it may mean receiving therapy from one discipline only. These reviews provide little information on how interventions from several disciplines were arranged to complement each other. Little analysis of synergism or antagonism of interventions has been undertaken.

Costs: there appear to be no reviews which consider the cost effectiveness of rehabilitation. This reflects the lack of health economic input into primary research. The authors of some reviews have speculated about the cost of the intervention under review but this appears to have been a *post hoc* approach which ignores the complexity of estimating the overall value of the cost and benefits of rehabilitation. Studies should aim to determine the components of the rehabilitation process which contribute to health care costs and which assist in the development of cost effectiveness methodology. A framework for this needs to be defined which should apply to many of the conditions and situations where rehabilitation takes place.

Limitations of the evidence

Aside from the methodological and research failings which are discussed in the next section, there are five important weaknesses in the evidence as presented.

Active components: little attempt has been made to identify the positive or active components of interventions which may have led to benefit.

Time scale: the majority of studies in the reviews were short term (<3 months) and this creates uncertainty about the potential longer term benefits of those interventions.

Social care: little appears to be known about the role of social care in isolation or as part of a co-ordinated package of care. Nothing appears to be known about the role of the boundary between health and social care in relation to the effectiveness of rehabilitation.

Transferability: there appears to be little information about the transfer of interventions from a hospital into a community. This is particularly important for many health systems and future research should consider the role and effectiveness of rehabilitation interventions in the community hospital, in residential care or nursing homes, in day centres and day hospitals and in the patient's own home.

Environment: there is a great lack of information about the role of the environment in diminishing disability and handicap. This may be implicit in research into, say, stroke care, but has not been brought out. This consideration would extend to simple aids to daily living, such as architecture, lighting and the outside environment.

The research effort

In general, there has been enormous and apparently unsuspected research into rehabilitation. However, the quality of that research as evidenced in these reviews leaves a lot to be desired. Some simple measures could improve matters for the future.

Conditions covered: a limited number have been tackled. Although some conditions which might be considered as priorities have been reviewed, many others have not. Table 7 indicates the present coverage of the reviews in this report.

Outcomes used: the range of outcomes is generally inadequate. There is too much emphasis on service matters and patient impairment. Outcomes evidence on handicap and carer issues is generally lacking. There needs to be closer congruence between outcomes used in research and outcomes of relevance to patients and practitioners. Trends in the delivery of health care and shifting of resources to the community sector will require additional outcomes methods to enable carers and community-based services to assess the value and progress of rehabilitation. Patient-centred outcomes often require performance of an action under observation and may be thought of as objective. In the community, this may be more difficult to organise. Newer outcomes which consider the impact of rehabilitation on informal carers or spouses, although requiring formal assessment to be of greatest value, may need to be more subjective although self-assessment scales and questionnaires are being developed rapidly. Outcome development and evaluation are still in their infancy although more attention is being given to health economics and cost-effectiveness.

Defining interventions: there is a strong tendency in reporting results to ignore the details of interventions. This creates uncertainty about the efficacy of the individual components of a complex intervention and makes it difficult to reproduce a package of care that implements the findings of research. A standard language for describing the inputs in a package of care is required. Closer definition of interventions would also assist those implementing research to understand what it is they need to emulate. Studies of 'extended therapy' need to be established in several areas since only short-term interventions have been undertaken. This includes stroke. The span of research does not reflect all stages in the process of rehabilitation; in particular, with the exception of one key review on the care of older people, the role of assessment of need is largely absent. Finally, the research is mainly into secondary care which is increasingly out of step with the present health service.

Research credibility: a major issue appears to be credibility of research in rehabilitation and the likelihood of uptake. Interventions which have dominated rehabilitation during the last decade have centred on half-hearted attempts at physical reintegration of a patient/client in the environment (aids, appliances, etc), or at psychosocial rehabilitation (a bit of support or counselling, sporadic provision of carer's groups, etc), and feeble attempts at reversing impairments [Tallis R. 1996]. Readers of this report may be surprised at the scale of the research and the scope of available reviews. A variety of factors may underlie this common stance. There is a major definitional problem which inhibits searching, assembly of results and clear identification of the field. Second, much of the research has been found to be lacking in scientific quality; this may 'smear' the good research which has been carried out. Third, the research tradition amongst the professionals involved is uneven and disparate. Unfortunately, research in rehabilitation is often considered uninteresting, ill-defined and impossible to undertake This is often because rehabilitation is thought not to have a scientific framework, is not a single quantifiable entity, and it is difficult to demonstrate efficacy. Although health professionals involved in rehabilitation do recognise the importance of identifying and carrying out research on the effectiveness of their work, this may explain the medical approach to research as revealed in this report. For example, the qualitative methodologies that are gaining ground, particularly in relation to satisfaction, would not be seen as sound research. There is much to be said for improving the standard of research with tighter studies and methods designed to assess the efficacy of packages of care. There is also a need for health economic appraisal which, at present, is sadly lacking.

Chapter 7

Recommendations

Key points

- Three groups of recommendations about rehabilitation are provided relating to services at present, future development and future research.

- Services need to concentrate upon the rehabilitation needs of their local population, especially older people.

- Services need to respond to the issues of access, organisation and the distinctive phases of care.

- Services should at the very least use the evidence of the systematic reviews in this report concerned with cardiac rehabilitation, stroke rehabilitation, comprehensive assessment of older people and educational approaches.

- Services should consider the implications of the reviews and their application to rehabilitation in other clinical areas that require the organisation of multiple staff groups, multiple inputs, multiple phases and patient involvement.

- Services need a set of core procedures that can be used widely across specialities, disciplines, client groups, and settings of care. The role of IT may need to be exploited here.

- Future developments of rehabilitation in services should be evaluated, perhaps using clinical audit, in order to promote quality improvement in care.

- Future developments in rehabilitation should be supported by some mechanism of cross learning between different agencies and localities. This will allow greater diffusion of good practice and know-how.

- Future development of rehabilitation will require iteration between the research and service communities so that research gets used.

- Future development of rehabilitation requires more training and education, including the development of local clinical teams.

- Future research in rehabilitation would benefit from an agreed transparent approach to prioritisation shared between funding bodies.

Key points (*cont.*)

- Future rehabilitation research will require improvements in methodology and reporting particularly around standardisation of description of interventions and outcomes, for which the classifications in this report may provide a starting point.

- Future rehabilitation research should continue to use systematic review which adhere to high standards, since there will inevitably be disparate trials that need to be brought together to maintain and update our understanding of effectiveness.

Future services

As indicated so far, there are strong reasons for implementing existing knowledge and increasing the focus on rehabilitation, particularly amongst older people. In this section of the community, there is a major need for rehabilitation and the greatest potential for benefit. Opportunities to improve the health and quality of life of older people should be ignored no longer. There are three themes emerging from the reviews presented in this report. The importance of access is suggested although it has not been thoroughly tested; this is regarded, particularly in education and patient empowerment, and in assessment, such as geriatric assessment, as a 'doorway' to care. The second theme concerns the proper organisation of complex team-based care delivering multiple inputs, with the strong suggestion that organising a service to deliver on a specific topic is an effective approach. The third theme is less clear but involves awareness of the different phases of rehabilitation – assessment, setting of objectives, implementing care plans and reviewing them. This process is not made explicit in research although they are principles that are well recognised.

This report also suggests developing some generic clinical approaches to rehabilitation which can be applied across a range of conditions and situations where it may be required. These need to be useable across several clinical disciplines – nursing, medicine, occupational therapy, physiotherapy etc. Such a development would also be useful in improving the skills and care in general settings. A multi-professional framework is necessary to promote the core context of methodologies to be used in future studies.

Future development

The development of rehabilitation within the NHS should be evaluated in the context of quality improvement and cross-learning between local services. This might be best achieved through large-scale national clinical audit. An added benefit of this would be the potential to monitor the practice of rehabilitation over time, an ability which is sadly lacking at the moment. There is a need for close liaison and iteration between routine practice in all sectors and research. This could be expressed by listing the priorities of research needs. It would also require collaboration on the use of harmonised outcome measures in research and practice since this would promote the easier understanding of research results by clinicians and managers.

Future development will also require a greater emphasis on training and education in rehabilitation. This is an important finding and links with growing awareness that for many involved in the process of rehabilitation, there is a distinct lack of both. This should begin at university with a recognised core content for each course offered additionally at a postgraduate facility. Since the operation of teams is seen as a key prerequisite for effective rehabilitation, consideration needs to be given to team development and maintenance in routine clinical care.

Future research

Greater focused coverage and prioritisation would probably help research, along with higher quality of description of interventions and outcomes used. Classifications developed for this report could be tested and developed further to meet this new language. The other issue to consider is the testing of complex interventions and the role of more sophisticated research designs, particularly when the effects of simple interventions may be small. A major challenge will be allowing long follow-up periods to be considered. Little research has considered safety and harmful effects of rehabilitation. This may be related to the timing of the intervention (e.g. physiotherapy on spastic limbs in stroke care), but there is inadequate knowledge of how rehabilitation actually affects limbs. In addition, little is known of the effects of age and ageing on the responses to rehabilitation. Rehabilitation will vary according to the disciplines involved but a graded approach rather than an all-or-nothing block of therapy may prove more beneficial since healing and improvement is more likely to be staged.

Future meta-analyses which evaluate rehabilitation studies should adhere to an accepted methodological/analytical framework:

(1) add clinical trials that include multidisciplinary rehabilitation programmes irrespective of the disability being addressed;

(2) include other important outcomes apart from functional level and mortality such as quality of life and psychological well-being which may also have been measured;

(3) accept only study designs which are rigorous and involve both randomisation of treatment and the presence of a control group. This kind of approach will strengthen the findings and provide a more informed view of rehabilitation in the light of current health care reforms.

Chapter 8

Conclusion

Much is known about the positive effects of rehabilitation in a variety of situations. There is already a large research base but this is fundamentally inadequate. There are a number of significant challenges to implementation of what is known. A new clear focus on rehabilitation with greater clarity of definition, purpose and role could exploit existing information, galvanise the present forces for change, provoke a more coherent research effort and stimulate real improvements in service delivery. Any projects which attempt to implement new service development in rehabilitation should also have in-built evaluations linked to quality improvement and good practice exchange.

General references

Cochrane Collaboration. *The Cochrane Collaboration Handbook*. Oxford: Update Software, 1997.

Hopkins A. *Measuring the quality of medical care*. London: RCP, 1990.

Keir D, Rehabilitation – complex values of a limitless team. Squires A (ed). *Rehabilitation of Older People*. London: Chapman and Hall, 1996: 42–54.

NHS Centre for Reviews and Dissemination. *Undertaking systematic reviews of research and effectiveness*. York: University of York, 1996.

NHS Executive. *Promoting clinical effectiveness. A framework for action in and through the NHS*. London: Department of Health, 1996.

NHS Executive. *The annual report of the NHS Health Technology Assessment Programme 1997. Identifying questions, finding answers*. London: Department of Health, 1997.

Tallis R. Rehabilitation of the elderly in the 21st century. *Journal of the Royal College of Physicians* 1992; 26: 413–422.

Wade DT. Stroke rehabilitation and long term care. *Lancet* 1992; 339:791–793.

References for reviews

Abenhaim L, Bergeron AM. Twenty years of randomised clinical trials of manipulative therapy for back pain: a review. *Clinical and Investigative Medicine* 1992; 15: 527–535.

Agosti V. The efficacy of treatments in reducing alcohol consumption : a meta-analysis. *International Journal of the Addictions* 1995; 30: 1067–1077.

Aker PD, Gross AR, Goldsmith CG, Peloso P. Conservative management of mechanical neck pain: systematic overview and meta-analysis. *British Medical Journal* 1996; 313: 129–136.

Anderson R, Meeker WC, Wirick BE, Mootz RD, Kirk DH, Adams A. A meta-analysis of clinical trials of spinal manipulation. *Journal of Manipulative & Physiological Therapeutics* 1992; 15: 181–194.

Assendelft WJ, Koes BW, Knipschild PG, Bouter LM. The relationship between methodological quality and conclusions in reviews of spinal manipulation. *Journal of the American Medical Association* 1995; 274: 1942–1948.

Beckerman H, de Ble R, Bouter LM, Cuyper H, Oostendorp R. The efficacy of laser therapy for musculoskeletal and skin disorders: a criteria-based meta-analysis of randomised clinical trials. *Physical Therapy* 1992; 72: 483–491.

Beckerman H, Bouter LM, van der Heijden GJMG, de Ble RA, Koes BW. Efficacy of physiotherapy for musculoskeletal disorders: what can we learn from research? *British Journal of General Practice* 1993; 43: 73–77.

Bien TH, Miller WR, Tonigan JS. Brief interventions for alcohol problems: a review. *Addiction* 1993; 88: 315–335.

Bobbio M. Does post myocardial infarction rehabilitation prolong survival? A meta-analytic survey. *Giornale Italiano di Cardiologia* 1989; 19: 1059–1067.

Brown SA. Studies of educational interventions and outcomes in diabetic adults: a meta-analysis revisited. *Patient Education and Counselling* 1990; 16: 189–215.

Cameron I, Finnigan T, Madhok R, Langhorne P, Handoll H. *Effectiveness of co-ordinated multidisciplinary in-patient rehabilitation for elderly patients with proximal femoral fracture.* Cochrane Database of Systematic Reviews. Oxford: Update Software, 1997.

Carlson M, Fanchiang SP, Zemke R, Clark F. A meta-analysis of the effectiveness of occupational therapy for older persons. *American Journal of Occupational Therapy* 1006; 50: 89–98.

Cohen JE, Goel V, Frank JW, Bombardier C, Peloso P. Guilemin F. Group education interventions for people with low back pain: an overview of the literature. *Spine* 1994; 19: 1214–1222.

Devine EC. Effects of psychoeducational care for adult surgical patients: a meta-analysis of 191 studies. *Patient Education and Counselling* 1992; 19: 129–142.

Devine EC. Meta-analysis of the effects of psychoeducational care in adults with asthma. *Research in Nursing & Health* 1996; 19: 367–376.

Di Fabio RP. Efficacy of manual therapy. *Physical Therapy* 1992; 72: 853–864.

Di Fabio RP. Efficacy of comprehensive rehabilitation programs and back school for patients with low back pain: a meta-analysis. *Physical Therapy* 1995; 75: 865–878.

Evans RL, Dingus CM, Haselkorn JK. Living with a disability: a synthesis and critique of the literature on quality of life, 1985–1989. *Psychological Reports* 1993; 72: 771–777.

Evans RL, Connis RT, Hendricks RD, Haselkorn JK. Multidisciplinary rehabilitation versus medical care: a meta-analysis. *Society of Science Medicine* 1995; 40: 1699–1706.

Gadsby JG, Flowerdew MW. *The effectiveness of transcutaneous electrical nerve stimulation (TENS) and acupuncture-like transcutaneous electrical nerve stimulation (ALTENS) in the treatment of patients with chronic low back pain.* Cochrane Database of Systematic Reviews. Oxford: Update Software, 1997.

Gam AN, Johannsen F. Ultrasound therapy in musculoskeletal disorders : a meta-analysis. *Pain* 1995; 63: 85–91.

Glanz M, Klawansky S, Stason W, Berkey C, Shah N, Phan H. Biofeedback therapy in poststroke rehabilitation: a meta-analysis of the randomised controlled trials. *Archives of Physical Medicine & Rehabilitation* 1995; 76: 508–515.

Glanz M, Klawansky S, Stason W, Berkey C, Chalmers TC. Functional electrostimulation in poststroke rehabilitation: a meta-analysis of the randomised controlled trials. *Archives of Physical Medicine and Rehabilitation* 1996; 77: 549–553.

Greenhalgh PM. *Shared care for diabetes: a systematic review.* London: The Royal College of General Practitioners, 1994.

van der Heijden GJM, Beurskens AJH, Koes BA, Assendelft WJJ, de Vet HCW, Bouter LM. The efficacy of traction for back and neck pain: a systematic, blinded review of randomised clinical trial methods. *Physical Therapy* 1995; 75: 93–104.

Holloway F, Oliver B, Collins E, Carson J. Case management: a critical review of the outcome literature. *European Psychiatry* 1995; 10: 113–128.

Hurwitz EL, Aker PD, Adams AH, Meeker WC, Shekelle PG. Manipulation and mobilisation of the cervical spine: a systematic review of the literature. *Spine* 1996; 21: 1746–1759.

Jones AP, Rowe BH. *Bronchopulmonary hygiene physical therapy in chronic obstructive pulmonary disease and bronchiectasis.* Cochrane Database of Systematic Reviews. Oxford: Update Software, 1997.

Katon W, Gonzalez J. A review of randomised trials of psychiatric consultation – Liaison studies in primary care. *Psychosomatics* 1994; 35: 268–278.

Kelley G, Tran ZV. Aerobic exercise and normotensive adults: a meta-analysis. *Medicine & Science in Sports & Exercise* 1995; 27: 1371–1377.

Koes BW, Bouter LM, Beckerman H, van der Heijden GJ, Knipschild P. Physiotherapy exercises and back pain: a blinded review. *British Medical Journal* 1991; 302: 1572–1576.

Koes BW, Assendelft WJJ, van der Heijden GJ, Bouter LM, Knipschild PG. Spinal manipulation and mobilisation for back and neck pain: a blinded review. *British Medical Journal* 1991; 303: 1298–1303.

de Kruif, van Wegen YP, Erwin EH. Pelvic floor muscle exercise therapy with myofeedback for women with stress urinary incontinence: a meta-analysis. *Physiotherapy* 1996; 82: 107–113.

Kugler J, Seelbach H, Kruskemper GM. Effects of rehabilitation exercise programmes on anxiety and depression in coronary patients: a meta-analysis. *British Journal of Clinical Psychology* 1994; 33: 401–410.

Lacasse Y, Wong E, Guyatt GH, King D, Cook DJ, Goldstein RS. Meta-analysis of respiratory rehabilitation in chronic obstructive pulmonary disease. *Lancet* 1996; 348: 1115–1119.

Linden W, Stossel C, Maurice J. Psychosocial interventions for patients with coronary artery disease ; a meta-analysis. *Archives of Internal Medicine* 1996; 156: 745–752.

Mari JJ, Adams CE, Streiner D. *Family intervention for those with schizophrenia.* Cochrane Database of Systematic Reviews. Oxford: Update Software, 1997.

Marrs RW. A meta-analysis of bibliotherapy studies. *American Journal of Community Psychology* 1995; 23: 843–870.

Marshall M, Gray A, Lockwood A, Green R. *Case management for severe mental disorders.* Cochrane Database of Systematic Reviews. Oxford: Update Software, 1997.

Moreland J, Thomson MA. Efficacy of electromyographic biofeedback compared with conventional physical therapy for upper-extremity function in patients following stroke: a research overview and meta-analysis. *Physical Therapy* 1994; 74: 534–543.

Mullen PD, Mains DA, Velez Rl. A meta-analysis of controlled trials of cardiac patient education. *Patient Education and Counselling* 1992; 19: 143–162.

Mumford E, Schlesinger HJ, Glass GV *et al*. The effects of psychological intervention on recovery from surgery and heart attacks: an analysis of the literature. *Am J Public Health* 1982;72:141–51.

NHS Centre for Reviews and Dissemination. Preventing falls and subsequent injury in older people. *Effective Health Care* 1996.

NHS Centre for Reviews and Dissemination. Stroke rehabilitation. *Effective Health Care* 1996b.

O'Connor GT, Buring JE, Yusuf S, Goldhaber SZ, Olmstead EM, Paffenbarger RS jr, Hennekens CH. An overview of randomised trials of rehabilitation with exercise after myocardial infarction. *Circulation* 1989; 80: 234–244.

Oldridge NB, Guyatt GH, Fischer ME, Rimm AA. Cardiac rehabilitation after myocardial infarction. Combined experience of randomised clinical trials. *Journal of the American Medical Association* 1988; 260: 945–950.

Ottenbacher KJ, Jannell S. The results of clinical trials in stroke rehabilitation research. *Archives of Neurology* 1993; 50: 37–44.

Robey, RR. The efficacy of treatment for aphasic persons : a meta-analysis. *Brain and Language* 1994; 47: 582–608.

Schleenbaker RE, Mainous AG. Electromyographic biofeedback for neuromuscular re-education in the hemiplegic stroke patient – A meta-analysis. *Archives of Physical Medicine & Rehabilitation* 1993; 74: 1301–1304.

Smith K, Cook D, Guyatt GH, Madhavan J, Oxman AD. Respiratory muscle training in chronic airflow limitation : a meta-analysis. *American Review of Respiratory Disease* 1992; 145: 533–539.

Stroke Unit Trialists' Collaboration. *A systematic review of specialist multidisciplinary team (stroke unit) care for stroke inpatients.* Cochrane Database of Systematic Reviews. Oxford: Update Software, 1997.

Stroke Unit Trialists' Collaboration (1997b). Collaborative systematic review of the randomised trials of organised inpatient (stroke unit) care after stroke. *Br Med J* 1997;314: 1151–9.

Stuck, AE, Siu AL, Wieland GD, Adams J, Rubenstein LZ. Comprehensive geriatric assessment: a meta-analysis of controlled trials. *Lancet* 1993; 342: 1032–1036.

Thomas J, Cook DJ, Brooks D. Chest physical therapy management of patients with cystic fibrosis. A meta-analysis. *American Journal of Respiratory & Critical Care Medicine* 1995; 151: 846–850.

Thomas JA, McIntosh JM. Are incentive spirometry, intermittent positive pressure breathing, and deep breathing exercises effective in the prevention of postoperative pulmonary complications after upper abdominal surgery? A systematic overview and meta-analysis. *Physical Therapy* 1994; 74: 3–16.

Whurr R, Lorch MP, Nye C. A meta-analysis of studies carried out between 1946 and 1988 concerned with the efficacy of speech and language therapy treatment for aphasic patients. *European Journal of Disorders of Communication* 1992; 27: 1–17.

Appendix 1

MEDLINE search strategy to identify systematic reviews

#1:   (meta-analysis or review literature).sh.
#2:   meta-analy$.tw.
#3:   meta-anal$.tw.
#4:   meta-analysis.pt.
#5:   review, academic.pt.
#6:   case report.sh.
#7:   letter.pt.
#8:   historical article.pt.
#9:   review of reported cases.pt.
#10:   review, multicase.pt.
#11:   review literature.pt.
#12:   1 or 2 or 3 or 4 or 5 or 11
#13:   6 or 7 or 8 or 9 or 10
#14:   12 not 13
#15:   animal.sh.
#16:   human.sh.
#17:   15 not (15 and 16)
#18:   14 not 17
#19:   **subject search terms**
#20:   18

Appendix 2

Examples of subject headings and/or keywords used

rehabilitation
rehabilitation centres
speech therapy
physiotherapy
physical therapy
occupational therapy
activities of daily living
art therapy
bibliotherapy
dance therapy
early ambulation
music therapy
rehabilitation of hearing impaired
rehabilitation, speech and language
music therapy
rehabilitation, vocational
day centres
needs transfer
ortho-geriatrics
habitation
resettlement
meta analysis
systematic review
review, academic

Appendix 3

Search scope for current medical literature (health care of older people)

Priority

Acta Neuropathol
Age Ageing
Alzheimer Dis Assoc Disord
Am J Phys Med Rehabil
Am J Psychiatry
Arch Gen Psychiatry
Arch Neurol
Arch Phys Med Rehabil
Bone Miner
Br J Psychiatry
Br J Rheumatol
Calcif Tissue Int
Clin Exp Gerontol
Clin Geriatr Med
Clin Rehabil
Exp Gerontol
Geriatr Cardiol
Geriatr Inf Immunol
Gerontologist
Gerontology
Int J Geriatr Psychiatry
J Am Geriatr Soc
J Cereb Blood Flow Metab
J Gerontol
J Nerv Mental Dis
J Rheumatol
Metab Bone Dis Relat Res
Neurology
Rev Ger
Scand J Rehabil Med
Soc Sci Med
Stroke

Other

Am J Epidemiol
Am J Med
Am J Med Sci
Am J Physiol
Ann Clin Biochem
Ann Intern Med
Arch Intern Med
Asian Med J
Aust N Z J Med
Biochem J
Biochim Biophys Acta
Br J Pharmacol
Br Med J
ClinSci
Curr Ther Res
Dan Med Bull
Dtsch Med Wochenschr
Eur J Biochem
Eur J Clin Pharmacol
JAMA
J Biol Chem
J Chron Dis
J Clin Invest
J Pathol
Jpn J Med
J R Soc Med
Lancet
Med J Aust
Minerva Med
Nature
Nature Med
N Engl J Med
N Z Med J
Physiol Rev
Postgrad Med J
Presse Med
Prev Med
Proc Natl Acad Sci
Q J Med
Schweiz Med Wochenschr
Science

Appendix 4

Classification system and inventory of rehabilitation interventions

For whom? *Study population*	Why? *Purpose*	By whom? *Staff*	What? *Nature*	Where? *Setting*	When? *Timing/ Phase*
General	Patient outcomes	Individual disciplines	Assessment, organisation	Home	Acute
Problem specific	Carer outcomes	Teams	Medical treatment	Nursing home etc	Post acute
Age specific	Service outcomes	Units	Physical	Day care	Discharge
Other	Other	Organisations & training	Psychological	Hospital	Post discharge
		Others	Social	Other	Other
			Aids & appliances		
			Environment		
			Organisation, and goals		

Appendix 5

Classification system and inventory of outcomes for assessing the effectiveness of rehabilitation

Patient centred outcomes
- Impairment
- Disability (primary and secondary ADL, senses, and communication)
- Handicap (including mood/morale, quality of life)
- Pain
- Goal attainment
- Service satisfaction
- Mortality/morbidity

Carer orientated outcomes
- Carer strain/mental health
- Satisfaction

Service orientated outcomes
- Subsequent service use (health/social)
- Institutionalisation/place of domicile/discharge
- Length of stay (hospital, rehab programme)
- Cost
- Readmission

Appendix 6: Evidence table

Authors	I REPORT CHARACTERISTICS					II DESCRIPTION OF INTERVENTION			
	Year	Country of origin	Title	Review Type	Trials & design	Study population	INTERVENTION Nature	Staff	Setting	Timing/phase
Abenhaim L, Bergeron A M	1992	Canada	Twenty years of randomised clinical trials of manipulative therapy for back pain: a review	SR	Total 21 RCT 21	People with acute and chronic back pain	Spinal manipulation vs. various other interventions		
Agosti V,	1995	USA	The efficacy of treatments in reducing alcohol consumption: a meta-analysis	MA	Total 12 RCT 12	People with alcohol misuse Total 1720 Mean age 35-50 yrs	Interventions to reduce alcohol consumption including drug therapy, counselling & behavioural therapy vs.placebo and others.		
Aker P D, Gross A R, Goldsmith C H, Peloso P,	1996	Canada	Conservative management of mechanical neck pain: a systematic overview and meta-analysis	MA	Total 24 RCT 24	People with mechanical neck disorders causing pain Total > 1200 Age N/S	Conservative management (medication, physical medicine, manual treatment, education)	Various	
Anderson R, Meeker W C, Wirick B E, Mootz R D, Kirk D H, Adams A,	1992	USA	A meta-analysis of clinical trials of spinal manipulation	MA	Total 23 RCT 23	People with low back pain Total > 3000	Spinal manipulative therapy		

41

III OUTCOMES USED

Authors	PATIENTS OUTCOMES							CARER OUTCOMES	SERVICE OUTCOMES
	Impairment	Disability	Handicap	Morbidity/ mortality	Pain	Satisfaction	Other		
Abenhaim L, Bergeron A M	EMG Range of movement	Disability	Quality of life		Pain score				
Agosti V,							Alcohol intake		
Aker P D, Gross A R, Goldsmith C H, Peloso P,					Pain scores				
Anderson R, Meeker W C, Wirick B E, Mootz R D, Kirk D H, Adams A,	Range of movement	Disability	Return to work		Pain score		Global assessment of recovery		

42

Authors	IV FINDINGS		
	Results	Authors conclusions	Comment
Abenhaim L, Bergeron A M	See Authors conclusions	Short-term positive benefits of manipulative therapy observed.	Longer term benefits need to be determined. Standardised measures / outcomes required.
Agosti V,	Reduced alcohol intake	In the short term and 1 year follow up studies, patients in the experimental group drank less than the control group. When the results were pooled, regardless of the follow up assessment periods, the experimental group drank less that controls.	Most effective treatments not identified. Comparisons of pharmacotherapy and psychosocial therapy needed. Common outcome criteria needed.
Aker P D, Gross A R, Goldsmith C H, Peloso P,	Reduced pain with manual treatment	Not enough detail in studies reviewed to assess efficacy and effectiveness.	Further research needed to determine optimal treatment approaches.
Anderson R, Meeker W C, Wirick B E, Mootz R D, Kirk D H, Adams A,	See Authors conclusions	Spinal manipulation appears consistently more effective than other treatments for which comparisons have been made.	Future studies require standardised measures and treatment schedules.

43

Authors	Year	Country of origin	Title	Review Type	Trials & design	Study population	II DESCRIPTION OF INTERVENTION INTERVENTION Nature	Staff	Setting	Timing/phase
Assendelft W J, Koes B W, van der Heijden G J, Bouter L M,	1996	NL	The effectiveness of chiropractic for the treatment of low back pain: an update and attempt at statistical pooling	MA	Total 8 RCT 8	People with acute or chronic low back pain	Chiropractic vs. various usual therapies	Chiropracter		Acute or chronic
Beckerman H, de Bie R, Bouter L, Cuyper H J, Oostendorp RAB,	1992	NL	The efficacy of laser therapy for musculoskeletal and skin disorders: a criteria-based meta-analysis of randomised clinical trials	SR	Total 36 RCT 36	People with musculoskeletal and skin disorders Total 1704	Laser treatment vs. physical therapy or placebo			
Beckerman H, Bouter L M, van der Heijden GJMG, de Bie RA, Koes B W,	1993	NL	Efficacy of physiotherapy for musculoskeletal disorders: what can we learn from research?	SR	Total 180 RCT 80	People with musculoskeletal disorders	Physiotherapy (including spinal manipulation, traction, exercise, ultrasound and laser therapy)			
Bien T H, Miller W R, Tonigan J S	1993	USA	Brief interventions for alcohol problems: a review	SR	Total 32 CCTs 32	People with alcohol problems (variously identified) Total 5951 Mean age 16-57	Brief interventions (usually advice and feedback) vs. no treatment and extended therapy			Post acute 3-120 months

III OUTCOMES USED

| Authors | PATIENTS OUTCOMES | | | | | | | CARER OUTCOMES | SERVICE OUTCOMES |
	Impairment	Disability	Handicap	Morbidity/ mortality	Pain	Satisfaction	Other		
Assendelft W J, Koes B W, van der Heijden G J, Bouter L M,	Spinal mobility	Back pain functional status	Quality of life		Pain score		Recovery		
Beckerman H, de Bie R, Bouter L, Cuyper H J, Oostendorp RAB,			Sport participation Sick leave		Pain score		Unspecified		
Beckerman H, Bouter L M, van der Heijden GJMG, de Bie RA, Koes B W,	Strength	Mobility Stability Functional status			Pain score				
Bien T H, Miller W R, Tonigan J S,	GGT levels						Alcohol intake Drinking behaviour Alcohol related problems		

45

Authors	IV FINDINGS		
	Results	Authors conclusions	Comment
Assendelft W J, Koes B W, van der Heijden G J, Bouter L M,	Insufficient data for pooling	No convincing evidence of benefit observed	Serious flaws in study designs and diversity of outcome measures prevents firm conclusions. Further research may be required.
Beckerman H, de Bie R, Bouter L, Cuyper H J, Oostendorp RAB,	No pooling	Weak evidence only for benefit with Laser Therapy.	Poor methodological quality of many studies reviewed. Better designed CRTs required.
Beckerman H, Bouter L M, van der Heijden GJMG, de Bie RA, Koes B W,	No pooling	No definite conclusions can be drawn owing to low methodological quality of the studies.	Larger trials of better quality are needed to establish efficacy of physiotherapy for musculoskeletal disorders.
Bien T H, Miller W R, Tonigan J S,	Pooling not performed	Provides support for efficacy of brief interventions in targeting drinking behaviour. There is encouraging evidence that the course of harmful alcohol use can be effectively altered by well designed intervention strategies.	Most effective interventions need more description and evaluation. Brief versus extended approaches require further study. Screening in health, social and employment systems needed.

46

Authors	I REPORT CHARACTERISTICS						II DESCRIPTION OF INTERVENTION			
	Year	Country of origin	Title	Review Type	Trials & design	Study population	INTERVENTION Nature	Staff	Setting	Timing/phase
Bobbio M	1989	Italy	Does post myocardial infarction rehabilitation prolong survival? a meta-analytic survey	MA	Total 10 RCT 10	People who have had a myocardial infarction Total 2300 Age range 25-71 years	Exercise programme			Mainly post acute
Brown SA	1990	USA	Studies of educational interventions and outcomes in diabetic adults: a meta-analysis revisited	MA	Total 82 RCT 32 CCT28	People with IDDM or NIDDM Total c.5000 Age range 11-92 years	Patient education	Usually multidisciplinary	Mixed - mainly clinic	Follow up 0-156 weeks
Cameron I, Finnegan T, Madhok F, Langhorn P, Handoll H.	1997	Australia	Effectiveness of co-ordinated multidisciplinary inpatient rehabilitation for elderly patients with proximal femoral fracture	CR	Total 6 CCT & QRCT 6	Older people with fracture of proximal femur which has been surgically treated Total 1143 patients Mainly >65 years	Co-ordinated rehabilitation	Supervised by geriatrician	Geriatric-orthopaedic rehabilitation unit (GORU) or other specialised multidisciplinary in patient rehabilitation	Post acute
Carlson M, Fanchiang SP, Zemke R, Clark F.	1996	USA	A meta-analysis of the effectiveness of occupational therapy for older persons	MA	Total 15 RCT 6 Other 9	Older people (in nursing homes or hospitals in 8 trials) Mean age 63-86 years	Occupational therapy		Nursing homes and hospitals (8 trials) Other settings (7 trials)	

Authors	III OUTCOMES USED								
	PATIENTS OUTCOMES							CARER OUTCOMES	SERVICE OUTCOMES
	Impairment	Disability	Handicap	Morbidity/ mortality	Pain	Satisfaction	Other		
Bobbio M,		Functional state		Death Recurrence					
Brown SA	Metabolic control Psychological status						Knowledge Self care behaviour Coping strategies		
Cameron I, Finnegan T, Madhok R, Langhorne P, Handoll H.		Functional status (Barthel & Katz scores)	Quality of life	Morbidity Death				Burden Stress	LOS Institutional care Support after discharge Cost
Carlson M, Fanchiang SP, Zemke R, Clark F.	Physical health Psychosocial well being	ADL							

48

Authors	IV FINDINGS		
	Results	Authors conclusions	Comment
Bobbio M	Reduced total mortality Reduced cardiac mortality	In only one study was the number of cardiac deaths significantly reduced in the trained patients.	Several CRTs of cardiac rehabilitation have been published since 1989. A revised meta-analysis may be warranted.
Brown SA	See Authors conclusions	Patient education in diabetes care is effective in producing positive patient outcomes especially in knowledge and metabolic control.	Supports these approaches as a routine part of diabetes care. Details of randomisation limited. Elderly patients require further study.
Cameron I, Finnegan T, Madhok E, Langhorne P, Handoll H.	See Authors conclusions	The question of effectiveness of different types of co-ordinated inpatient rehabilitation after proximal femoral fracture cannot be answered conclusively. There is a trend to effectiveness when combined outcome variables are considered.	Further studies are needed paying particular attention to methodological issues and should aim to establish the effectiveness of multidisciplinary rehabilitation overall rather than attempting to evaluate its components.
Carlson M, Fanchiang SP, Zemke R Clark F.	See Authors conclusions	Occupational therapy in a global sense is effective in achieving important outcomes in the older population	Further research needs to address which therapeutic approaches work best with older patients in order to achieve specific types of therapeutic outcomes

Authors	I REPORT CHARACTERISTICS						II DESCRIPTION OF INTERVENTION			
	Year	Country of origin	Title	Review Type	Trials & design	Study population	INTERVENTION		Setting	Timing/phase
							Nature	Staff		
Cohen J E, Goel V, Frank J W, Bombardier C, Peloso P, Guilemin F	1994	Canada	Group education interventions for people with low back pain	SR	Total 13 CCT 9	People with low back pain (acute 3 studies, chronic 9 studies, unspecified 1 study) Mean age 28-51 years	Group education inter-ventions (including , exercise training and physiotherapy) vs.	N/S	Mixed	Up to 18 month follow up
Devine E C,	1996	USA	Meta-analysis of the effects of psychoeducational care in adults with asthma	MA	Total 31 RCT 31	People with asthma Total 1860 Mean age 25-50 years	Psychoeducational care (education, behavioural skill development, cognitive therapy and/or nonbehavioural support/counselling) vs. usual care		Mixed (mainly outpatient treatment)	
Devine E C,	1992	USA	Effects of psychoeducational care for adult surgical patients: a meta-analysis of 191 studies	MA	Total 191 (60% CRTs)	People undergoing abdominal or thoracic surgery Mean age 29-76 years	Psychoeducational and pain control (including use of health care information, skills teaching, psychosocial support)		Hospital	Pre and post operative

III OUTCOMES USED

Authors	PATIENTS OUTCOMES							CARER OUTCOMES	SERVICE OUTCOMES
	Impairment	*Disability*	*Handicap*	*Morbidity/ mortality*	*Pain*	*Satisfaction*	*Other*		
Cohen J E, Goel V, Frank J W, Bombardier C, Peloso P, Guilemin	Spinal mobility	Functional status	Sick leave		Pain score		Knowledge of condition		
Devine E	Respiratory function		Well being	Asthma attacks			Knowledge of condition Compliance Use of PRN medication		Use of health care
Devine E C,	Mood Anxiety Distress			Complications	Pain		Use of analgesics Use of sedatives		LOS

Authors	IV FINDINGS		
	Results	Authors conclusions	Comment
Cohen J E, Goel V, Frank J W, Bombardier C, Peloso P, Guilemin F,	No statistical pooling of results	At 1 year follow up, no evidence in the 6 quality studies of clinically important benefits in any of the measures outcomes.	Insufficient evidence to recommend group education for patients with low back pain.
Devine E C,	Reduced asthmatic attacks Improved respiratory volume Improved peak flow rate Improved functional status Improved functional status Improved adherence/knowledge Improved use of PRN medication remedication regime Improved psychological well being	Education and relaxation based behavioural interventions improve clinical benefits in adult asthmatics	Future research needs to include both random assignment to treatment condition and a placebo type control treatment.
Devine E C,	See Authors conclusions	Some beneficial effects are seen with psychoeducational approaches in the treatment of recovery, post surgical pain and psychological distress.	Tabulated data on outcomes not provided. Nurses were the major providers of this care. The increasing trend towards day surgery and admission on morning of operation may alter relevance of these approaches.

52

Authors	**I REPORT CHARACTERISTICS**						**II DESCRIPTION OF INTERVENTION**			
	Year	Country of origin	Title	Review Type	Trials & design	Study population	INTERVENTION			Timing/phase
							Nature	Staff	Setting	
Di Fabio F P,	1992	USA	Efficacy of manual therapy	SR	Total 14 CCT 10	People with somatic pain syndromes and associated disability — Total >1400 — Most <65 years	Manual therapy (manipulation or mobilisation)			Acute, sub acute or chronic (> 8 weeks)
Di Fabio F P,	1995	Canada	Efficacy of comprehensive rehabilitation programs and back school for patients with low back pain: a meta-analysis.	MA	Total 19 RCT 19	People with acute, subacute and chronic back pain — Total 2373 — Mean age 42 years	Back school +/- comprehensive rehabilitation		Mainly outpatient	
Evans R L Dingus C M, Haselkorn J K,	1993	USA	Living with disability: a synthesis and critique of the literature on quality of life 1985-1989	SR	Total 8 RCT 8	People with disability — Total 2297	Very mixed (including drugs, surgery, rehabilitation, nursing, medical care, hospice care)		In patient	
Evans R L Connis R T, Hendrick R D, Haselkorn J K,	1995	USA	Multidisciplinary rehabilitation versus medical care: a meta-analysis	MA	Total 11 RCT 9 Other 2	People with a need for rehabilitation — Total 2183 — Mean age 75 years	Multidisciplinary rehabilitation for 2 weeks to 3 months vs. conventional medical care		In patient	

Authors

III OUTCOMES USED

Authors	PATIENTS OUTCOMES							CARER OUTCOMES	SERVICE OUTCOMES
	Impairment	Disability	Handicap	Morbidity/ mortality	Pain	Satisfaction	Other		
Di Fabio R P,		ADL Depression			Pain score				
Di Fabio R P,	Spinal motion Strength Endurance	Disability	Quality of life Work		Pain		Education Compliance		
Evans R L, Dingus C M, Haselkorn J K,			Quality of life						
Evans R L, Connis R T, Hendricks R D, Haselkorn J K		Functional ability	Return to residence				Death		

Authors | IV FINDINGS

Authors	Results	Authors conclusions	Comment
Di Fabio F P,	See Authors conclusions	Clear evidence of effectiveness of manipulation for low back pain.	Trials needed on manual therapy for peripheral joints. Better descriptions of treatment interventions and measures of compliance and on designing studies with equivalent interventions.
Di Fabio F P,	See conclusions	Back school with comprehensive rehabilitation is more effective than back school alone. Pain and physical impairment showed greatest improvement but work and disability outcomes did not improve.	Further research on the role of back school in preventing chronic pain and identifying what factors improve work/vocational outcomes needed. What changes in the health care system are needed to improve results in work related injury?
Evans R L Dingus C M, Haselkorr J K,	No statistical pooling of results	Poor research design. Little reliable objective data to inform decision makers about improvements in quality of life after rehabilitative care for disabled population.	More quality studies needed on quality of life including more uniform and valid criteria.
Evans R L Connis R T, Hendrick R D, Haselkorr J K,	Improved survival Improved function while in hospital Improve home return rate	At discharge MD care led to improved survival and functional ability with an increased chance of returning home. Effects not sustained for survival and functioning.	Extended effects of MD care in home and post acute care settings needs evaluation. Other outcomes (e.g. behavioural) should be employed in future studies.

Authors	I REPORT CHARACTERISTICS						II DESCRIPTION OF INTERVENTION			
							INTERVENTION			
	Year	Country of origin	Title	Review Type	Trials & design	Study population	Nature	Staff	Setting	Timing/phase
Gadsby JG, Flowerdew MW.	1997	UK	The effectiveness of transcutaneous electrical nerve stimulation (TENS) and acupuncture -like transcutaneous electrical nerve stimulation (ALTENS) in the treatment of patients with chronic low back pain	CR	Total 6 RCT 6	People with chronic lower back pain for at least 8 weeks duration Total 288 (mean age 45-50 years)	TENS & ALTENS			
Gam A N, Johannsen F,	1995	Denmark	Ultrasound therapy in musculoskeletal disorders: a meta-analysis	MA	Total 22	People with various musculoskeletal diseases Total 1953	Ultrasound treatment vs. sham treatment, other treatment and non treatment			
Glanz M, Klawansky S, Stason W, Berkey C, Chalmers T C,	1996	USA	Functional electrostimulation in post-stroke rehabilitation: a meta-analysis of the randomised controlled trials	MA	Total 4 RCT 4	People with a stroke Total 132 Mean age 56-59 years	Functional electrostimulation vs. control		Academic rehabilitation medicine settings	Post acute (1-29 months post stroke)
Glanz M, Klawansky S, Stason W, Berkey C, Shah N, Phan H, Chalmers T C,	1995	USA	Biofeedback therapy in post-stroke rehabilitation: a meta-analysis of the randomised controlled trials	MA	Total 8 RCT 8	People with a stroke and arm and leg weakness Total 168 Age N/S	Biofeedback therapy		Academic rehabilitation medicine settings	Post acute (2-45 months post stroke)

III OUTCOMES USED

Authors	PATIENTS OUTCOMES							CARER OUTCOMES	SERVICE OUTCOMES
	Impairment	Disability	Handicap	Morbidity/ mortality	Pain	Satisfaction	Other		
Gadsby JG, Flowerdew MW.	Range of movement	Functional status	Return to work		Validated pain score		Side effects		
Gam A N, Johannsen F,	Range of motion Grip strength	Walking distance functional capacity			Pain score		Use of analgesics X-Ray findings		
Glanz M, Klawansk~ S, Stason W, Berkey C, Chalmers T C,	Muscle force								
Glanz M, Klawansky S, Stason W Berkey C, Shah N, Phan H, Chalmers T C,	Joint range of motion								

Authors	IV FINDINGS	
	Results	Comment
Gadsby JG, Flowerdew MW,	See Authors conclusions	TENS appears to reduce pain and improve the range of movement in chronic low back pain subjects	A definitive randomised controlled study of ALTENS, TENS, placebo/no treatment controls is needed to confirm these findings.
Gam A N, Johannsen F,	No evidence of effectiveness	There is a lack of substantial support for ultrasound in the treatment of musculoskeletal disorders.	Future studies need to resolve the question whether ultrasound can supplement exercise therapy in well designed placebo controlled studies. Better designed studies and more explicit descriptions of methods are needed.
Glanz M, Klawansky S, Stason W, Berkey C, Chalmers T C,	Increased muscle force	Pooling from randomised trials support FES as promoting muscle recovery after stroke. This effect is statistically significant. There is a reasonable likelihood of clinical significance as well.	Results do not confirm functional improvement. Studies of sustained treatment required.
Glanz M, Klawansky S, Stason W, Berkey C, Shah N, Phan H, Chalmers T C,	No evidence of effectiveness	Does not support efficacy of biofeedback therapy in restoring range of motion.	Small sample sizes decreases the validity of the conclusions. Most effective timing of the intervention needs identifying.

58

| Authors | I REPORT CHARACTERISTICS | | | | | | II DESCRIPTION OF INTERVENTION | | | |
	Year	Country of origin	Title	Review Type	Trials & design	Study population	INTERVENTION Nature	Staff	Setting	Timing/phase
Greenhalgh PM,	1994	UK	Shared care for diabetes. A systematic review	SR	Total 24 RCT 5 CCT 5 Other 14	People with IDDM and NIDDM Total >2185 (1053 in CRTs)	Shared care		Interface between secondary and primary care	
der Heijden van G J M Beurskens AJH, Koes B W, Assendelft WJJ, de Vet HCW, Bouter LM,	1995	NL	The efficacy of traction for back and neck pain: a systematic, blinded review of randomised clinical trial methods	MA	Total 21 RCT 17	People with back or neck pain	Traction vs. Conservative treatment or placebo			
Holloway F, Oliver N, Collins E, Carson J,	1995	UK	Case management : a critical review of the literature	MA	Total 23 RCT 10 CCT 4 Other 9	People with varying degrees of mental illness inc schizophrenia. Total >3803 (mainly <65 yrs).	Case management (including Assertive Community Treatment, direct care and brokerage models) vs. standard community care or hospital admission	Individuals and interdisciplinary teams		Follow up 3-60 months
Hurwitz L, Aker P D Adams A H, Meeker W C, Shekelle G,	1996	USA	Manipulation and mobilisation of the cervical spine	MA	Total 67 RCT 14	People with subacute or chronic neck pain	Cervical spine manipulation and mobilisation vs. usual care	GP, chiropracter, manual therapist, physical therapist, physiotherapist, medical doctor		Subacute & chronic

III OUTCOMES USED

Authors	Impairment	Disability	Handicap	Morbidity/ mortality	Pain	Satisfaction	Other	CARER OUTCOMES	SERVICE OUTCOMES
	PATIENTS OUTCOMES								
Greenhalgh PM,	Glycosylated haemoglobin Complications recorded			Death		Satisfaction	Data recording Costs		Review frequency Lab test frequency Hospital referrals
der Heijden van G J M, Beurskens AJH, Koes B W, Assendelft WJJ, de Vet HCW, Bouter LM,	Spinal mobility	Functional status			Pain score		Global measure		
Holloway F, Oliver N, Collins E, Carson J,	Mental state		Quality of life Social functioning			Satisfaction	Medication compliance Attendance	Family burden	LOS Admissions Use of services Costs
Hurwitz E L, Aker P D, Adams A H, Meeker W C, Shekelle P G,				Headache	Pain score				

Authors	IV FINDINGS	
	Results	Comment
Greenhalgh PM,	See conclusions	Long-term follow up of patients in RCTs of shared care systems are needed to establish that acceptable outcomes are maintained over time. Cost effectiveness studies are also needed.
der Heijden van G J M, Beurskens AJH, Koes B W, Assendelf WJJ, de Vet HCW, Bouter LM,	No evidence of effectiveness	Further trials needed with explicit descriptions of methodological features and important outcomes. Development of a credible traction placebo needed.
Holloway F, Oliver N, Collins E, Carson J,	Decrease in bed days Improved service satisfaction Improved engagement with service Improved social functioning	The "effective" elements of case management need to be identified. Better designed studies providing a health economic evaluation are required.
Hurwitz L, Aker P D Adams A H, Meeker C, Shekelle G,	Reduced pain Reduced headache	Better randomised studies forcusing on the frequency and duration of treatment are needed to clarify the effectiveness of various doses of therapy. Cost effectiveness studies also required.

Authors conclusions:

Results show a lack of structure in diabetes care in general practice and a lack of systematic preparation by the hospital team when patients are discharged to GP care. Recommended level of care is outlined.

Methodological flaws in design of studies means no clear conclusions can be reached about efficacy of traction for patient with back / neck pain. Studies were of small sample size (usually <100).

Case management (especially direct care) reduces number and length of hospital admissions

Cervical spine manipulation and mobilisation provide short term benefits for some patients with neck pain and headache. Although the complication rate of manipulation is small, the potential for adverse outcomes must be considered.

Authors	I REPORT CHARACTERISTICS						II DESCRIPTION OF INTERVENTION			
							INTERVENTION			
	Year	Country of origin	Title	Review Type	Trials & design	Study population	Nature	Staff	Setting	Timing/phase
Jones AP, Rowe BH	1997	USA	Bronchopulmonary hygiene physical therapy in chronic obstructive pulmonary disease and bronchiectasis	CR	Total 10 RCT 10	People with chronic obstructive pulmonary disease and bronchiectasis (mean 41-72 yrs) Total 153	Postural drainage or Postural drainage and percussion			
Katon W, Gonzalez J,	1994	USA	A review of randomised trials of psychiatric consultation–liaison studies in primary care	SR	Total 11 RCT 7	People referred to the consultation liaison psychiatry service Total 2718 Age ??	Consultation liaison psychiatry		Primary care	
Kelley G, Tran Z V,	1995	USA	Aerobic exercise and normotensive adults: a meta-analysis	MA	Total 35 RCT 14 CCT 6 NT 15	People with normal blood pressure Total 1076 Mean age range 35-45 years	Aerobic exercise			Treatment 1-21 months
Koes B W, Assendelft W J, van der Heijden G J, Bouter L M, Knipschild P G,	1991	NL	Physiotherapy exercises and back pain a blinded review	SR	Total 35 RCT35	People with back or neck pain Total >4000	Spinal manipulation and mobilisation			

62

Authors	III OUTCOMES USED										
	PATIENTS OUTCOMES									CARER OUTCOMES	SERVICE OUTCOMES
	Impairment	Disability	Handicap	Morbidity/ mortality	Pain	Satisfaction	Other				
Jones AP, Rowe BH	Dyspnoea Forced vital capacity Respiratory rate Arterial oxygen tension CHR resolution Presence of dysrythmias										LOS
Katon W, Gonzalez J,	Mental health					Satisfaction					Medical treatment Costs Doctor behaviour
Kelley G, Tran Z V,	BP (diastolic and systolic - standard measurement) Heart rate						Body mass index				
Koes B W, Assendelft W J, van der Heijden G J, Bouter L M, Knipschild P G,	Joint range of movement	Functional status			Pain score		Improvement Drug use				Use of services

63

Authors	IV FINDINGS		
	Results	Authors conclusions	Comment
Jones AP, Rowe BH		Given the size and quality of the trials, the research on BHPT is, at best, confusing. The routine application of BHPT to patients with chronic airways obstruction cannot be supported on the basis of this evidence	There is a need to conduct an adequately sized RCT that examines the effects of BHPT on clinical outcomes related to morbidity and mortality.
Katon W, Gonzalez J,	See conclusions	Unclear: Inadequate discussion of findings prevents firm conclusions.	Further RCTs may be required to investigate area further.
Kelley G, Tran Z V,	See conclusions	Aerobic exercise reduces resting systolic and diastolic blood pressure in normotensive adults.	Future studies with full reporting of blood pressure measurement techniques; information on adherence rate of subjects and exercise programs are necessary.
Koes B W, Assendelft W J, van der Heijden G J, Bouter L M, Knipschild P G,	See Authors conclusions	Efficacy of spinal manipulation has not been proven although manipulation may be effective in certain sub groups of patients with back / neck pain.	Better methodological quality of trials needed

Authors	| I REPORT CHARACTERISTICS						II DESCRIPTION OF INTERVENTION			
	Year	Country of origin	Title	Review Type	Trials & design	Study population	INTERVENTION Nature	Staff	Setting	Timing/phase
Koes B W, Bouter L, Beckerman H, van der Heijden G J, Knipschild P G,	1991	NL	Spinal manipulation and mobilisation for back and neck pain: a blinded review	SR	Total 16 RCT 16	People with acute or chronic low back pain	Physiotherapy exercises			
de Kruif Y, van Wegen EEH	1996	NL	Pelvic floor muscle exercise therapy with myofeedback for women with stress urinary incontinence: a meta-analysis	MA	Total 10 RCT 4 CCT 2 Other 4	Women with stress incontinence (except for one man) Total 758 (8 trials with less than 35 subjects) All ages in 5 trials >55 years in 4 trials	Pelvic floor exercises & myofeedback			
Kugler J, Seelbach H, Kruskemper GM,	1994	Germany	Effects of rehabilitation exercise programmes on anxiety and depression in coronary patients: a meta-analysis	MA	Total 15 CCT 15	People with ischaemic heart disease	Exercise programmes focusing on anxiety and depression			1-48 months
Lacasse Y, Wong E, Guyatt G H, King D, Cook DJ, Goldstein RS	1996	Canada	Meta-analysis of respiratory rehabilitation in chronic obstructive pulmonary disease	MA	Total 14 RCT 13	People with Chronic Obstructive Pulmonary Disease Total 468 (mean age 60-73 yrs)	Exercise training with or without education and psychological support for at least four weeks		Mixed - mainly home based	Follow up 6-30 months

III OUTCOMES USED

Authors	PATIENTS OUTCOMES							CARER OUTCOMES	SERVICE OUTCOMES
	Impairment	Disability	Handicap	Morbidity/ mortality	Pain	Satisfaction	Other		
Koes B W, Bouter L, Beckerman H, van der Heijden G J, Knipschild P G,	Joint range of movement	Mobility ADL			Pain score		Improvement		
de Kruif YP, van Wegen EEH	Continence diary Constraction force Bladder stress								
Kugler J, Seelbach H, Kruskemper GM,	Psychological state (various scores)								
Lacasse Y, Wong E, Guyatt GH, King D, Cook DJ, Goldstein RS	Exercise capacity		Quality of life						

Authors	IV FINDINGS	
	Results	Comment
	Authors conclusions	
Koes B W, **Bouter L,** **Beckerman H,** **van der Heijden G J,** **Knipschild P G,**	See Authors conclusions Exercise therapy not proven as effective or non-effective.	Further trials of good methodology quality needed.
de Kruif YP, **van Wegen EEH**	See Authors conclusions Reduction in incontinence in 5 trials (including 2 controlled trials) and increase in contraction force in 5 trials (including 3 controlled trials)	Further RCTs required. Longer periods of therapy needed. Benefits in older patients require clarification.
Kugler J, **Seelbach H,** **Kruskemper GM,**	See Authors conclusions Exercise alone is not the optimal treatment for emotional disturbances in coronary patients.	More studies needed on patients who psychosocially benefit and those who deteriorate after exercise.
Lacasse Y, **Wong E,** **Guyatt GH,** **King D,** **Cook DJ,** **Goldstein RS**	See Authors conclusions Respiratory rehabilitation relieves breathlessness and improves control over COPD. The value of this improvement is not clear. Respiratory rehabilitation is an effective part of care in patients with COPD.	Clinical benefit was apparent providing some justification for promoting pulmonary rehabilitation.

Authors	I REPORT CHARACTERISTICS						II DESCRIPTION OF INTERVENTION			
							INTERVENTION			
	Year	Country of orgin	Title	Review Type	Trials & design	Study population	Nature	Staff	Setting	Timing/phase
Linden W, Stossel C, Maurice J,	1996	Canada	Psychosocial interventions for patients with coronary artery disease	MA	Total 23 RCT 23	People with Coronary artery disease Total 3180	Various pyschosocial interventions (for example psychotherapy, counselling, education, exercise, etc.) vs. standard rehabilitation	Mixed (doctor, nurse, educator, lay)		
Mari JJ, Adams CE, Streiner D	1997	UK	Family intervention for schizophrenia	CR	Total 12 RCT and QRCT 12	People with Schizophrenia and/or schizoaffective disorders (standardised diagnosis) Total >686 (not specified in one study) Age range 15-65 years (mainly <40 years)	Family psychosocial Interventions including creating alliances with relatives who care for patients, reducing adverse family atmosphere, problem solving and reduction of guilt/anger by family		Not restricted to inpatient care	Follow up 6-96 months
Marrs R W,	1995	USA	A meta-analysis of bibliotherapy studies	MA	Total 79 Uncertain designs	People working on their concerns Total 4677 Mean age 35 years	Bibliotherapy/reading programmes vs. control and therapist administered treatments		Home	
Marshall M, Gray A, Lockwood A, Green R.	1997	UK	Case management for severe mental disorders	CR	Total 9 RCT/QRCT 9	People with severe mental illness Total 1540 Mean age generally <40 years	Case management (including Assertive Community Treatment) vs. standard community care or hospital admission		Community	

III OUTCOMES USED

Authors	PATIENTS OUTCOMES							CARER OUTCOMES	SERVICE OUTCOMES
	Impairment	Disability	Handicap	Morbidity/ mortality	Pain	Satisfaction	Other		
Linden W, Stossel C, Maurice J.	Psychological state Blood pressure Pulse Lipids			Mortality Non fatal cardiac events					
Mari JJ, Adams CE Streiner D	Mental state (several measures) Relapse			Suicide Death					Hospital admission
Marrs R W,	Weight Behaviour Psychological state						Compliance		
Marshall M, Gray A, Lockwood A, Green R.	Mental state Psychological well being		Quality of life Social functioning Self esteem	Death Suicide		Patient satisfaction	Number of needs	Carer satisfaction	Need assessment Care planning Contact maintenance Hospital admission Costs Imprisonment

69

Authors	IV FINDINGS		
	Results	Authors conclusions	Comment
Linden W, Stossel C, Maurice J,	Reduced psychological distress Reduced SBP Reduced HR Reduced cholesterol level Decreased mortality Decreased cardiac recurrence rate	Intervention led to greater reductions in psychological distress, BP, HR, cholesterol; 41% and 46% declines in mortality and cardiac events at 2 years.	Recommends inclusion of psychosocial treatment in cardiac rehabilitation; further research to define most effective form of this intervention.
Mari JJ, Adams CE, Streiner D	See Authors conclusions	Families receiving this intervention may expect the member with schizophrenia to relapse less, be in hospital less, but that the family burden and levels of emotion expressed to remain the same.	The number needed to treat (e.g. for relapse at one year = 65) may be more acceptable to clinicians and families than to purchasers and providers of care.
Marrs R W,	See Authors conclusions	Bibliotherapy is effective for certain problem types - assertion training, anxiety and sexual dysfunction.	Only 5 studies reported reading ability of the participants, and only 14 reported educational level. Too few studies adequately reported how much the participants used the bibliotherapy for that variable to be analysed.
Marshall M, Gray A, Lockwood A, Green R.	See Authors conclusions	Case management moderately increases a severely mentally ill person's chance of being reliably followed up in the community. It approximately doubles the number of hospital admissions with little evidence of causing an improvement in mental state.	Further research on CM approaches are unlikely to be needed. New approaches to CM are required using validated instruments.

Authors	I REPORT CHARACTERISTICS					II DESCRIPTION OF INTERVENTION			
	Year	Country of origin	Title	Review Type	Trials & design	Study population	INTERVENTION		Timing/phase
							Nature	Staff	Setting	
Moreland, Thomson M A,	1994	Canada	Efficacy of electromyographic biofeedback compared with conventional physical therapy for upper-extremity function in patients following stroke: a research overview and meta-analysis	MA	Total 6 RCT 6 (Outcome data in 5 only)	People with a stroke and arm dysfunction. Age range 19-89 years	Electromyographic feedback for 2-11 weeks vs. usual physiotherapy)		Hospital or rehabilitation centre	Post acute (2-416 weeks post stroke)
Mullen P D, Mains D A, Velez R,	1992	USA	A meta-analysis of controlled trials of cardiac patient education	MA	Total 38 RCT c.14 CCT 28	People with Coronary artery disease Total c.5000 Mean age 50-60 years)	Cardiac education and psychosocial interventions	Various	Various	Post acute follow up 0-48 months
Mumford E, Schlesinger HJ, Glass GV	1982	USA	The effects of psychological intervention on recovery form surgery and heart attacks: an analysis of the literature	MR	Total 34	People recovering from surgery and myocardial infarction	Psychological intervention	Various		Post-acute
NHS Centre for Reviews and Dissemination	1996	UK	Preventing falls and subsequent injury in older people	SR	Total 36 RCT/QRCT 36 Home exercise 23 Home assess. 9	People with falls and falls risk Total >11,000 Aged >60 years in all but one study	A variety of preventive measures including Exercise Home assessment/surveillance Shoes Dietary interventions Hip protectors			Follow up 1-48 months

71

Authors — III OUTCOMES USED

Authors	PATIENTS OUTCOMES							CARER OUTCOMES	SERVICE OUTCOMES
	Impairment	Disability	Handicap	Morbidity/ mortality	Pain	Satisfaction	Other		
Moreland J, Thomson M A,	Muscle force Range of motion EMG findings	Arm function (various measures)							
Mullen P D, Mains D A, Velez R,	Exercise Diet BP Stress		Return to work	Morbidity Death			Drug compliance Smoking		
Mumford E, Schlesinger HJ, Glass GV	Physiological indicators			Post op complications	Pain rating		Treatment co-operation Drug use		Recovery speed LOS
NHS Centre for Reviews and Dissemination	Balance Postural control Muscle strength Risk factors for falls			Falls Injuries			Home safety changes		

IV FINDINGS

Authors	Results	Authors conclusions	Comment
Moreland , Thomson M A,	No significant benefit	Results do not conclusively indicate superiority of either therapy. The estimated effect size is small.	Therapists should consider other factors, such as cost or patient preference, before advising which treatment is given. Acute and chronic cases need separate study.
Mullen P D, Mains D F, Velez R,	See Authors conclusions	Interventions led to measurable impacts on BP, mortality, exercise and diet	Details of randomisation were vague. Calls for "individualised" programmes to be set up, involving carers if possible. Community post-acute studies needed.
Mumford E, Schlesinger HJ, Glass GV	See Authors conclusions	Beyond the intrinsic value of offering humane and considerate care, the evidence is that psychological care can be cost effective.	Further research required.
NHS Centre for Reviews and Dissemination	See Authors conclusions	Limited evidence only of benefit for any single intervention.	More studies needed to confirm relevance and acceptability to UK health care system, including cost effectiveness studies.

Authors	I REPORT CHARACTERISTICS						II DESCRIPTION OF INTERVENTION			
	Year	Country of origin	Title	Review Type	Trials & design	Study population	INTERVENTION			Timing/phase
							Nature	Staff	Setting	
NHS Centre for Reviews and Dissemination	1992	UK	Stroke rehabilitation	SR	Total 17 RCT 14	People with a stroke	Rehabilitation vs. usual care		Mixed -mostly hospital	
O'Connor G T, Buring J E, Yusuf S, Goldhaber S Z, Olmstead E M, Paffenbarger R S Jnr, Hennekens CH,	1989	USA	An overview of randomised trials of rehabilitation with exercise after myocardial infarction	MA	Total 22 RCT 22	People after myocardial infarction Total 2554 Most < 65 years	Rehabilitation with exercise vs. usual care, advice, and low intensity exercise			Post acute (Follow up 1-5 years)
Oldridge N B, Guyatt G H, Fischer M E, Rimm A A,	1988	USA	Cardiac rehabilitation after myocardial infarction. Combined experience of randomised controlled clinical trials	MA	Total 10 RCT 10	People after myocardial infarction Total 4347 Mean age 53-55 years	Cardiac rehabilitation (exercise and/or risk factor management)			Post acute (2-9 months, follow up 24-60 months)
Ottenbacher KJ, Jannell S,	1993	USA	The results of clinical trials in stroke rehabilitation research	MA	Total 36 Various	People with a stroke Total 3717 Mean age 69 years	Stroke rehabilitation			Post acute (mean 7 weeks post stroke)

74

Authors	III OUTCOMES USED							CARER OUTCOMES	SERVICE OUTCOMES
	PATIENTS OUTCOMES								
	Impairment	Disability	Handicap	Morbidity/ mortality	Pain	Satisfaction	Other		
NHS Centre for Reviews and Dissemination	Neuromuscular deficit Depression	ADL Communication Gait	Quality of life Social functioning	Death			Complications	General health	LOS Onset of therapy Place of discharge Follow up arrangements Later hospital use
O'Connor G T, Buring J E Yusuf S, Goldhaber S Z, Olmstead E M, Paffenbarger R S Jnr, Hennekens CH,				Death Morbidity					
Oldridge N B, Guyatt G H, Fischer M E, Rimm A E,				Death Recurrence					
Ottenbacher KJ, Jannell S,	Motor reflex function Cognitive skill Visual perception	Lang ability ADL							LOS

75

Authors	IV FINDINGS		
	Results	Authors conclusions	Comment
NHS Centre for Reviews and Dissemination	No statistical pooling performed	Some evidence that formal rehabilitation after stroke is effective and best provided by well organised multidisciplinary teams. Enough evidence to suggest that therapy services should be provided in hospitals and community settings.	Larger trials of good methodological quality using a range of validated outcome measures are needed to clarify stroke rehabilitation care.
O'Connor G T, Buring J E, Yusuf S, Goldhaber S Z, Olmstead E M, Paffenbarger R S Jnr, Hennekens CH,	Reduced mortality Reduced reinfarction	Cardiac rehabilitation programs with exercise reduce risk of death by 20%. Reduced risks of cardiovascular mortality and fatal infarction persist for at least 3 years after infarction.	A larger RCT is required to establish if the "physical" component of cardiac rehabilitation has independent effects.
Oldridge N B, Guyatt G H, Fischer M E, Rimm A A,	Reduced death rate Reduced cardiac death rate	For appropriately selected patients, comprehensive cardiac rehabilitation results in a significantly lower fatal event rate, although not non-fatal reinfarction.	Quality of life and cost effectiveness studies required.
Ottenbacher KJ, Jannell S,	Improved function	Focused stroke rehabilitation given early is effective (especially in younger patients).	Need for more RCTs to be established with better defined patient entry criteria, treatment modalities and using clinically important outcome measures.

Authors	I REPORT CHARACTERISTICS						II DESCRIPTION OF INTERVENTION			
	Year	Country of origin	Title	Review Type	Trials & design	Study population	INTERVENTION			Timing/phase
							Nature	Staff	Setting	
Robey R R	1994	USA	The efficacy of treatment for aphasic persons: a meta-analysis	MA	Total 21 CCT 4	People with aphasia (mainly due to stroke)	Rehabilitation for aphasia (various types of speech therapy)	Speech and Language therapists and lay people		
Schleenbacker R E, Mainous F G,	1993	USA	Electromyographic biofeedback for neuromuscular re-education in the hemiplegic stroke patient: a meta-analysis	MA	Total 8 RCTs & CCTs 8	People with a stroke and hemiplegia Total 192	Electromyographic biofeedback for 2-3 weeks vs. physiotherapy or no treatment			Post acute
Smith K, Cook D, Guyatt G H, Madhavan J, Oxman A D,	1992	Canada	Respiratory muscle training in chronic airflow limitation: a meta-analysis	MA	Total 17 RCT 17	People with chronic airflow limitation	Respiratory muscle training			
Stroke Unit Trialists' Collaboration	1996	UK	A systematic review of specialist multidisciplinary team (stroke unit) care for stroke inpatients)	CR	Total 12 RCT/QRCT 12	People with a stroke	Specialist multidisciplinary team care vs. usual general medical ward care	Multi disciplinary stroke care team	Stroke Unit in hospital	Post acute

Authors	III OUTCOMES USED									CARER OUTCOMES	SERVICE OUTCOMES
	PATIENTS OUTCOMES										
	Impairment	Disability	Handicap	Morbidity/ mortality	Pain		Satisfaction		Other		
Robey R R,	Speech (Boston Diagnostic Aphasia Examination and other measures)	Index of communicative ability									
Schleenbacker R E, Mainous A G,	Grasp, grip and pinch	Gait pattern Need for walking aids									
Smith K, Cook D, Guyatt G H, Madhavan J, Oxman A D,	Respiratory muscle strength Pulmonary function	Functional capacity	Respiratory quest								
Stroke Unit Trialists' Collaboration				Death							LOS Institutional care

Authors	IV FINDINGS	
	Results	Authors conclusions	Comment
Robey R R	See Authors conclusions	The outcomes witness the clear superiority in performance of persons receiving treatment by a speech language pathologist	Lack of randomisation and heterogeneity of studies reduces the impact (validity) of this meta analysis.
Schleenbaker R E, Mainous A G,	Increased function	EMG biofeedback appears to be a useful therapy increasing function for hemiplegic stroke patients	Small sample sizes limits interpretation of findings. Includes 2 studies reviewed and 1 study excluded in Ref 33 (used different outcomes). Larger randomised studies required.
Smith K, Cook D, Guyatt G H, Madhavar J, Oxman A D,	See Authors conclusions	Little evidence for respiratory muscle training treatment for patients with chronic airflow limitation.	Resistance training programmes warrant further study.
Stroke Unit Trialists' Collaboration	See Authors conclusions	Stroke patients managed within speciality stroke units are more likely to be alive and living at home a year after stroke than those managed on general medical wards. Time in hospital not prolonged	Research needed to identify which aspects of stroke unit care beneficial and generalisable. Formal measures of functional ability should be included in future studies.

Authors	I REPORT CHARACTERISTICS						II DESCRIPTION OF INTERVENTION			
							INTERVENTION			
	Year	Country of origin	Title	Review Type	Trials & design	Study population	Nature	Staff	Setting	Timing/phase
Stroke Unit Trialists' Collaboration	1997	UK	Collaborative systematic review of the randomised trials of organsied inpatient (stroke unit) care after stroke	MA	Total 19 RCT 17 QRCT 2	People who have had a stroke Total 3247 Age range not stated	Organised in-patient (stroke unit) care vs. conventional care	Medical, nursing, physiotherapy, occupational therapy, speech therapy and social work	Hospital	Acute and subacute
Stuck A E, Siu A L, Wieland G D, Adams J, Rubenstein L Z,	1993	Switzerland USA	Comprehensive geriatric assessment: a meta-analysis of controlled trials	MA	Total 28 CCT 28	Older people receiving care in a variety of settings Total 9871	Comprehensive Geriatric Assessment		Five settings	Varied (Follow up 6-36 months)
Thomas J A, McIntosh J M,	1994	USA	Are incentive spirometry, intermittent positive pressure breathing and deep breathing exercises effective in the prevention of postoperative pulmonary complications after upper abdominal surgery? A systematic overview and meta-analysis	MA	Total 14 RCT 14	People undergoing abdominal or thoracic surgery Total 1337 Age range 29-76 years	Breathing Interventions including Incentive spirometry (IS), Deep breathing exercises (DBE), and Intermittent positive pressure breathing (IPPB)		Hospital	Post operative
Thomas J, Cook D J, Brooks D,	1995	Canada	Chest physical therapy management of patients with cystic fibrosis	MA	Total 35 RCTs 35	People with cystic fibrosis aged > 5years	Chest physical therapy (7 different combinations)			Treatment for up to three years

III OUTCOMES USED

Authors	PATIENTS OUTCOMES							CARER OUTCOMES	SERVICE OUTCOMES
	Impairment	Disability	Handicap	Morbidity/ mortality	Pain	Satisfaction	Other		
Stroke Unit Trialists' Collaboration		ADL		Death					LOS Institutional care
Stuck A E, Siu A L, Wieland G D, Adams J, Rubenstein L Z,		Function Cognitive function	Home living	Mortality					Hospital admission
Thomas J A, McIntosh J M,	chest X ray Physical examination Pulm function tests Blood gases Cough/dyspnoea Pyrexia			Post op pulmonary complication					
Thomas J, Cook D J, Brooks D,	Pulmonary function tests (FEV1)						Sputum weight		

81

IV FINDINGS

Authors	Results	Authors conclusions	Comment
Stroke Unit Trialists' Collaboration	Long term reduction in death and death/dependency independent of patient age, sex, stroke severity, and types of organisation	Organised stroke care resulted in long term reductions in death, dependency and the need for institutional care. The observed benefits were not restricted to any particular subgroup of patients. No systematic increase in use of resources (LOS) apparent	Excellent in depth systematic review showing the benefits of organisation of care
Stuck A E, Siu A L, Wieland G D, Adams J, Rubenstein L Z,	More living at home Reduced mortality Improved function (GEMU) Improved cognitive function (GEMU & IGCO)	CGA programs linking geriatric evaluation with strong long-term management are effective for improving survival and function in older people.	Processes of CGA need to be refined in order to enhance its effectiveness.
Thomas J A, McIntosh J M,	Reduced pulmonary complications	IS, DBEx and IPPB equally effective in preventing post-operative lung complications and each more effective than no physical therapy.	Further research on frequency and optimal dosage of treatment should be standardised before effectiveness can be determined.
Thomas J, Cook D J, Brooks D,	Improved sputum production Improved pulmonary function	Standard physiotherapy resulted in a significantly greater sputum expectoration than no treatment. STX with STD is associated with a moderate statistically significant increase in FEV over STD alone.	Future studies need to be randomised, double blind, to maximise internal validity and of sufficient power to minimise random error. Patient characteristics need to be described clearly.

Authors

Whurr R, Lorch M P, Nye C

I REPORT CHARACTERISTICS

Year	Country of origin	Title	Review Type	Trials & design	Study population
1992	UK/USA	A meta-analysis of studies carried out between 1946 and 1988 concerned with the efficacy of speech and language therapy treatment for aphasic patients	SR	Total 166 RCT 55	People with aphasia Total 1336 Mean age 62 years

II DESCRIPTION OF INTERVENTION

INTERVENTION			
Nature	Staff	Setting	Timing/phase
Speech and language therapy (various types, for a mean of 28 weeks)		Mainly hospital and clinic	Mainly post acute

III OUTCOMES USED

PATIENTS OUTCOMES								CARER OUTCOMES	SERVICE OUTCOMES
Impairment	Disability	Handicap	Morbidity/mortality	Pain	Satisfaction	Other			
Psychological state	Speech and language (various assessments)								

IV FINDINGS

Results	Authors conclusions	Comment
See Authors conclusions	Efficacy of speech and language therapy is inconclusive due to a lack of data on dependant variables.	Further research needed conforming to RCT design for measurement of disorder, measurement tools employed and clear details of the treatment program.